Male, Unknown
C.J. GRIFFITHS

NO EXIT PRESS

First published in the UK in 2025 by No Exit Press,
an imprint of Bedford Square Publishers Ltd,
London, UK

noexit.co.uk
@noexitpress

ISBN
978-1-83501-300-7 (Paperback)
978-1-83501-301-4 (eBook)

2 4 6 8 10 9 7 5 3 1

Typeset in 11 on 13.4pt Adobe Garamond Pro
by Avocet Typeset, Bideford, Devon, EX39 2BP
Printed and bound in Great Britain by
CPI Group (UK) Ltd, Croydon CR0 4YY

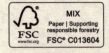

The manufacturer's authorised representative in the EU for product safety is
Easy Access System Europe, Mustamäe tee 50, 10621 Tallinn, Estonia
gpsr.requests@easproject.com

To Laura, Will and Eleanor, with all my love.

Prologue
ICU

He hears a voice in the darkness. Deep and confident.
'What's his name, nurse?'

The shuffling of notes. A pause. The next voice is female. Brusque, efficient.

'Unknown, doctor.'

The male voice becomes louder, taking on the firm, prescriptive tone of the medical professional talking to the sedated patient.

'Sir, I'm Doctor Morris. You're in intensive care. We need to insert a tube to help you breathe.'

But he already knows where he is and what is happening to him. He is calm; he understands that hearing is always the last of the senses to disappear. He can picture the room; the sterile walls, the banks of screens with their coloured lines tracing pulses, ECGs, oxygen saturations, carbon dioxide levels. He can almost smell the chlorhexidine, can imagine the alarms and the crash calls, the whine of the defibrillators, the flat, drumming sound of theatre shoes hitting the floor as staff run towards another cardiac arrest. They won't be working on him though, not for a while at least. He has planned too carefully for that.

Perhaps he will hear her voice soon. He needs to hear it.

As Morris continues quietly in his slow, public school monotone, he tries to picture him. Tall and thin. Hatchet-faced. Humourless but professional.

'How much propofol in this syringe, nurse?'

'A hundred milligrams, doctor.'

'What does he weigh?'

'Seventy-two kilograms. He's an alcoholic, by the way. His LFTs are terrible.'

'Mental health issues as well, by the looks of it. Doctor Carter will need to be informed. Just another twenty IV, please.'

He feels himself drifting. He rides the wave. As long as she finds him, as long as he gets the message to her, everything will finally be all right.

'Okay, let's have a look. Pass me the laryngoscope.' Then, louder, 'Just relax, sir. Everything's fine.'

He thinks of her as she was when he first knew her. He wonders what she looks like now. As his thoughts spiral into the past and the anaesthetic begins to work, he feels his muscles relax.

She will come.

Later he sleeps, but it's not sleep as he used to know it. Voices continue to float in and out of his consciousness until it's impossible to tell where dreaming stops and real voices begin. There is no pain. He has no urge to breathe. The regular hiss of the ventilator punctuates everything in a soft background wave of noise like the slow rush of shingle on a wide, sloping beach. A small circular bay. A waterfall. He chases the memory, but the rest is lost in time. Maybe they were both there once; perhaps it was where they hunted for shells and skimmed stones together. Maybe the *shhhh* of the ventilator is nothing but the comforting movement of the sea upon the earth.

He doesn't know when she'll come, but he is certain she will. He has been in hell. She has to come.

Time flows, indeterminate. Then a voice, impossibly distant.

'Edie. Look what this guy has done to himself.'

He feels no surprise, only warmth. At last, she is here. He speaks, silently.

Edie. It's been so long.

And all of this is for you.

1

Edie

'Why don't you call in sick? Come back to bed.'

The varnished floorboards are cold as I swing my feet out from under the warm covers. My breath carries wisps of condensation in the grey light of early morning. Harry's suggestion is beyond tempting; I can feel the soft touch of his hand on my back, moving across my t-shirt, finding its way underneath, brushing my skin. I let it happen for a moment, eyes closed, then glance at my phone. Six-fifteen. Shuffling free, I grab my dressing gown. The manic babble of a disc jockey bursts out of my old clock radio as the ten-minute snooze ends. Harry wriggles across the bed under the duvet, then a hand snakes out and slams the off button. Only his tousled dark hair is visible as he groans. I turn the clock radio upright again.

'Hey, that was a present from my mum. You'll break it.'

I can just hear the muffled voice from under the covers. 'Edie, come back to bed. Say the car wouldn't start or something.'

Leaning down, I kiss the top of his head and pull my dressing gown tight. 'For a doctor, you have a really slack work ethic.'

His face appears. His grey eyes are lidded, still sleepy. 'Ah, but I'm a psychiatrist. I can rationalise anything. Wanting to stay in bed and make love rather than go to work is technically a coping mechanism.'

'Coping mechanism? What do you need to cope with, precisely?'

'My undying lust for you,' he replies, propping himself on his elbow and wrapping his arm around my waist.

'Good answer,' I laugh, twisting from his grip. 'But the department is short-staffed, so your issues will have to keep.'

9

I skitter to the bathroom on the balls of my feet and start the shower, letting it run hot and the steam gather before stepping in. Turning my face to the jet of water, I blast away the headache loitering on the edges of my temples that reminds me I had a couple of glasses too many last night. It's shocking what a busy shift can do to your willpower. I let my thoughts drift towards work, hoping that nothing too taxing has come into the unit overnight. Halfway through rubbing shampoo into my hair, I remember that Morris is the consultant this week. I breathe slowly and deeply in the steam, willing the headache to disappear. I can deal with Richard Morris and I can deal with a hangover, but not in the same shift.

My eyes are closed against the jet of water rinsing the last of the shampoo suds when I hear the shower door snick open and closed with a quick waft of cool air. Then I feel Harry's chest pressed against my shoulders and his lips brushing the back of my neck. I relax my body into his, catching the lingering traces of last night's aftershave on him before the water washes it away. His touch feels good, and he'd managed to come in at the perfect time to make it a welcome surprise. Wiping my eyes, I half-twist to face him as water runs from his hair and onto my cheek, his hands moving across my stomach and encircling my waist. Our eyes meet, blinking in the steam.

'Well, showering together is good for the environment.' Harry smiles. Our lips touch, and the remnants of the hangover are finally forgotten.

Half an hour later I can hear him clattering downstairs in the kitchen as I finish getting ready. I've always been amazed at how low-maintenance Harry is; his grooming regime consists of towel-drying his hair, dragging a comb through it, then a quick blast of body spray. He throws his clothes on at random and somehow still manages to look as if he made an effort. He has been in the kitchen for fifteen minutes by the time I get downstairs; enough time to make coffee and French toast. This is fast and easy for him; he's fallen into the role of chef automatically and is a natural cook, from quick breakfasts to dinner party menus. He's one of those people who never measures anything but always seems to get the balance right. From the moment we moved in together a year ago I was happy for the kitchen to be his domain. I can mix anaesthetic drugs and calculate complicated doses in my head, but I have no talent whatsoever near a stove and would probably burn water.

Harry slides two pieces of toast onto my plate, pushes it across to me, and pours out a large mug of coffee.

'Hey, Edes. Don't forget about tonight.'

Tonight? Oh God, the future in-laws. I've yet to work out whether their attitude towards me is genuine disdain or just my imagination; a symptom of the insidious impostor syndrome that began in medical school. 'I'm really sorry, Harry, I can't make it. I'm going to be finishing late tonight. I've got a session with Doctor Wilson.' I feel a small pang of guilt as I see Harry's smile fade and realise that I'd looked a little too pleased to have an excuse not to go. I can sense him watching me as I eat, can feel him wanting to talk. The interrupted conversation is like a deep breath being held, but if we started on his family now we might not stop. 'I'm sorry, okay? I'll call you later.'

'Yeah.' He pauses. 'You know, you could always talk to me about things, rather than that quack Wilson. I love you. I want to help.'

He looks at me in a way that always used to make me feel transparent. His eyes searching, encouraging, a look designed to enable dialogue. It can be unnerving until you realise it is just a body language technique. Smoke and mirrors from Psychiatry 101. I'm sorry, Harry, but if I don't get to go there, neither do you.

'I sometimes wonder if going out with a shrink was a wise move?' I say, wincing as I swallow the hot coffee. I pick up the second piece of toast to eat on the go and grab my bag and hoodie. 'Maybe you just see me as a project?'

'Of course not. It was love at first sight, that's all,' he calls after me. 'You know I've always had a thing for Daisy Ridley.'

'I look nothing like Daisy Ridley.' I feign indignation, but can't hide my smile.

Harry notices and smiles too. His insistence on my resemblance to the actress had been a standing joke since we'd watched *The Marsh*

King's Daughter on one of our early dates. But despite pretending to be indifferent, I'd been secretly delighted at the compliment as I'd watched her dark hair, angular face and feline hazel-green eyes. It had done wonders for my self-esteem. A lesson on how to rid yourself of insecurity by proxy.

Harry's smile fades and he becomes serious, cajoling. 'Listen, Edes, the meal isn't until eight. It's my father's birthday; they've got people coming up from London.'

'So they can show off their Warwickshire mansion instead of the *pied à terre* in Chelsea?' I take the car keys from the hook by the kitchen door. 'Are you ready? I'll give you a lift?'

'Yeah.' He puts the plates into the sink. 'You know something? If I didn't know better, I'd say you've got a chip on your shoulder. You're an inverted snob. There must be *something* you like about my family.'

'Of course,' I say, and grin. 'The look on their faces when I drop my aitches at dinner parties.'

Shaking his head, Harry pulls the front door shut behind us.

2
Harry

The King George is a sprawling modern hospital twenty minutes' drive east from our rented terrace in an unfashionable part of Harborne. It is one of those hospital sites that's spread exponentially over the years, with wide car parks and modern steel and glass blocks towering over the original, rust-coloured Victorian buildings, which cluster in the corner of the site near the main entrance. We arrive at seven-thirty, so there are plenty of spaces left in the staff car park, and, after we've pecked goodbye, I head towards the older part of the site and the Psychiatric Department. As I walk, I watch the hospital coming to life; ambulances are moving in and out of the emergency bays, staff are arriving, and people with puzzled frowns are crawling along in their cars as they try to decipher the blue department signs.

The large Gothic entrance to the Psychiatry Department is behind a perimeter wall with an ornate nineteenth-century archway, which marked the boundary of the old hospital. Apparently, this original building used to be a Victorian asylum. It's still imposing, like a nineteenth-century prison, but the old buildings only accommodate our office space now. The main unit and secure section are in a modern PFI build attached to it. When I first arrived here, I thought the staff would recognise the irony of the building's history, but most didn't. Many of my colleagues at the KG are the most humourless, strait-laced bunch I've ever met, although thankfully one or two are easier to get along with. One of my favourites is outside in the smoking corner of the courtyard lighting a cigarette, her hand cupped.

Smiling, I wander over to say hello.

13

'Morning, Beth.'

Taking a large drag, she blows the smoke upwards and away from me in that polite gesture some people do when around friends who don't smoke. Her soft voice has a strong Highlands burr. 'Ah, Harry. Good morning.'

Doctor Beth Lafferty is a singular, intense woman in her fifties, who trained in Edinburgh and has since done the rounds in a variety of mental health hospitals and units. She left university with a first-class degree and not an ambitious bone in her body. While all her sharp-elbowed contemporaries, and the young climbers like me, clambered up the ladder, she happily stagnated on the same rung for years. She is the least affected person I've ever known, and one of the few people who I immediately got on with when I arrived at the King George. She won't take credit for it, but she is partly responsible for getting Edie and me together. Two years ago, when Morris originally referred Edie for sessions, I was allocated her as a client. But I had seen her around the hospital and before the first consultation I'd sat down with Beth and begged her for advice. I knew I was going to have a conflict of interest. On my side at least, the attraction to Edie was immediate and overwhelming. Her condition only made her more interesting, her insecurities more intriguing. Beth had laughed softly, surprisingly unfazed, and talked me through the ethics of the psychiatrist–client relationship, things I already knew but had never faced in practice. Finally, she said she'd reallocate Edie to Amy Wilson; that if she wasn't officially my patient then there was no ethical conflict. So go ahead and ask her out, Harry, she'd said, smiling, adding, young love is a wonderful thing. Just don't get involved in her case.

On the day I waited for Edie outside the department with the intention of asking her for a drink, I was shaking with nerves. You know when that chemistry is right, and the stakes felt higher than they ever had with any previous relationship. When she'd agreed to go out with me, my usual self-sabotaging tendency kicked in and I'd done my best to blow it by arranging a series of dates that, in hindsight, should have made her run a mile. They were more like activities at kids' parties: bowling, cinema, pizza parlours, that sort of teenage thing. I should have looked for gallery exhibitions and museums or something. But somehow, instead of seeing me as a guy in a worrying state of arrested development, she sensed something in me worth sticking with, a spark worth kindling. I felt it too, and we hit it off straight away, talking for hours about nothing in particular and, within a few weeks, sharing things more personal.

But the spanner was about to be thrown in the works. I hate to admit it to myself, but Edie is right about my family. They're cold towards her, particularly my father, and I don't know why. I admit that my parents can be hard people to like sometimes, and I say that as a dutiful son. They are often kind, generous and sweet. But they can also be controlling, elitist and judgemental. Beth is looking at me as she smokes, a wry smile on her face.

'A penny for them, Harry.'

'Ah, don't worry. Just thinking about my family. That's probably why I look grim.'

'Oh dear. Family.' Beth stubs her cigarette out on a nearby wall and throws the butt into a bin. She has no guilt about smoking in public as some people do, which makes me like her more. She's old-school and doesn't care what anyone thinks of her. 'Good job I don't have one; they're more trouble than they're worth.'

I smile. 'My parents are having a party tonight and I want Edie to come. I'm determined for them to know how serious we are.'

'What you mean is you want your father to know. The great professor?'

Blunt and incisive as always. She is nearly thirty years older than me, the same grade, and all her career has watched the rat race of the psychiatry world with amused detachment. She knows everything and everyone, and what she hasn't experienced personally she has heard about. She knows my father, although he wouldn't have a clue about her because, to him, she's one of the little people. She can't do anything for him, so why bother remembering her name?

'Yeah, I suppose. I want their approval. So what do I do?'

'You're engaged to her, Harry, so you persevere. I'm an old cynic, and even I think you make a lovely couple.' We walk into the building together, Beth's voice echoing in the wide polished-oak hallway. 'Stick with it, Harry. Edie is where your future lies, not your father. Be your own person. Your father will come around to the idea.'

'Thanks, Beth. I'll see you for a coffee later.'

She raises her hand briefly and peels off towards her office.

Stick with it. Edie is where your future lies.

That's what I'd hoped she'd say, and I know she's right.

3

Edie

After graduation, I'd always imagined living in a suitably cool part of London – Camden or Hoxton maybe – and working in a big, dynamic hospital. UCH would have done. St Thomas' at a push. London placements always attract us provincial trainees like moths, particularly those like me, who fought our way into medical school through sheer bloody-mindedness. Yet here I am, serving my anaesthetic training in the West Midlands, under the guidance of a mentor who treats me like I'm an interesting new biopsy sample. Harry landed on his feet with a residence at the Maudsley followed by a Clinical Fellowship at the KG and will almost certainly make consultant in three years. It's always useful being to the manner born, and doors do tend to fly open when your father is a professor at the Royal College of Psychiatrists. Okay, Harry, maybe I do have a chip on my shoulder.

Still, the upside of working at the King George is Jaz, my saviour. I'd often heard the blasphemous med school rumours that it's actually the nurses who teach specialist trainees most of what they know. For me, Jaz is the proof. Not only did she help me though a rocky first few months, saving me from making some basic mistakes and sparing my blushes, but she was always the one dragging me down to The Five Bells after a tough day and telling me gently – in exactly the way I needed to be told – that tough days in ICU are par for the course. Brooding alone is the worst thing anyone can do after a difficult shift, she'd said, and I won't allow it. And something would flicker in her eyes telling me she'd been there, and a similar thing in me responded. We are the same

17

age and technically I'm her senior, but with that look I knew it was time to listen to experience.

Harry and I peck a brief goodbye at the car before he makes his way towards the older part of the hospital where the Department of Psychiatry is based. His genial ambling gait never changes, whether he's late or early for work. He walks through the car park as though he's on a ramble through some woods on a day off, whereas I feel the work mask slip on as soon we drive through the main gates. One of Harry's most endearing traits is the way he manages to be both laid back and yet permanently fascinated with the world, as if he thinks he's always about to miss out on something. I watch him disappear around the corner of the Emergency Department, then I head towards the main hospital wing.

On the way in I swing past the High Dependency Unit to check on a patient, taking a quick diversion through the large rectangular grey block that houses most of the wards. As I buzz myself into the HDU I'm glad to see the patient I want to talk to is awake. Cath Saunders is an elegant woman in her mid-forties, and when I poke my head around the door of the unit she is sitting up in bed and chatting to the nurse who is checking her observations. A week ago she was with us downstairs in ICU on a ventilator, with the worst case of urosepsis I had seen in my brief clinical life. Every day her husband Mark and teenage daughter Jess had come in to sit by her bedside and hold her hand in a silent, loving vigil, which moved me every shift, as did their quiet, dignified relief when she turned the corner and her condition improved. I'd been asked by Morris to extubate her the day before, and to see her now sitting up and talking is exactly the start I'd hoped for this shift. I introduce myself again, but from her smile I know she remembers me. I don't admit that coming to see her was partly a selfish thing to do. It's an act of affirmation; a way of keeping positive and balancing the more difficult things about working in critical care.

We chat about her family for a while, then glancing at the clock near her bed I realise how time has slipped by. Wishing her the best, I head downstairs, rushing into the department at five to eight, tying my scrubs. Luckily, the morning handover hasn't started yet. One by one, staff are gathering, drifting towards the nurses' station as if by gravity, the early shift with mugs in their hand, the night shift counting the minutes until eight. As the desk gets busier, I scan the board. One new patient.

Male, unknown. Tricyclic toxicity.

There is a tug on my sleeve, and I turn to see a tall male nurse with a white t-shirt under his scrubs, his blond hair neatly side parted. Matt. He's rubbing his clipped beard. He grins at me; something has clearly happened. Matt thrives on gossip and drama.

'Edie, come with me.'

'Matt, you made me jump. Why is this patient down as an unknown male? If he's unidentified, shouldn't the ED have given him a randomly generated name?'

'Yeah, someone in ED obviously didn't get the memo.' Matt tugs my sleeve again. 'Never mind his name, just come here.'

'The handover's about to start.'

'It can wait. You seriously need to see this.' Matt pulls me towards the bays.

His eyes are glittering with impatience, his brow furrowed. Matt's a good nurse when he wants to be, but there seems to be no middle ground with him. At the moment he's at the excitable end of his spectrum. He drags me by the sleeve, towards a bay with the curtains pulled across.

'Matt. What are you doing?'

His voice is an urgent hiss. 'Shut up a minute. Look at this.'

Furtively, he pulls me behind the curtains. On the bed is a man whose age is hard to guess. Mid-fifties perhaps. His skin is sallow, with the light sheen and the yellow tinge of someone whose liver is failing. He is intubated. The ventilator hisses softly. Matt pulls the bed sheet down, exposing his chest.

'Edie, look what this guy has done to himself.'

The noises of the unit fade away as the writing, livid purple, swamps my consciousness. My vision narrows, so all of my sight is filled with it. Reality pauses, slides out of view. Some clinical, detached part of me wonders about the dedication, the patience, to perform this act of self-mutilation. I study his face. Nothing. Heart pounding, I search my memory, my early memory. The empty spaces. The things that are hidden.

I touch the wounds, trace the words carved across his skin. Some of the letters are infected, the result of a dirty blade, serous fluid oozing from the crudely drawn words, rosé pink. A single, jagged message.

My name. A plea.

Edie Carter. Forgive me.

4

Edie

Richard Morris has a habit of steepling his hands under his narrow chin while he's thinking. Sitting opposite me, he pauses for effect, his spidery fingers drumming against each other softly, his scrubs hanging loosely on angular shoulders. We watch each other in silence across his desk. His office is unwelcoming and sterile in the way only an office in a newly built hospital wing can be. He has tried in vain to personalise it – framed certificates line the wall, his family grin stiffly from a photo on the desk and pot plants wilt in the corners – but it still feels like a waiting room.

'So, how are you feeling, Edie?'

'I'm not sure. Worried.'

'I see. So do you recognise him?'

His abrupt manner makes me bristle. Okay, I wasn't expecting an arm around my shoulder; Morris doesn't do soft and fluffy. But given I'd spent the last hour in a state of blurred confusion, and my heart rate had only just returned to normal, a little more understanding might have been nice.

'No, I have no idea who he is, Doctor Morris.' Then, on a frustrated impulse, 'This has been quite a shock though. *Obviously.*'

I wouldn't have had the nerve to slip that sarcastic dig into my conversation a year ago. It takes a while at the start of a medical career for the sheen of politeness to wear off, for the realisation to sink in that you either fight your corner or you don't get taken seriously. If you're a woman, you fight even harder. Recently, I'd been embracing the *screw you* attitude of my teenage years; the hair-trigger sense of injustice that had propelled me from an underperforming state comprehensive to medical school. Confidence is self-perpetuating, or so I was always being told. And then this happens, to drag my insecurities from the deep hole I'd buried them in.

Morris's eyebrows lift a few millimetres, and a smile of sympathy finally touches his lips. 'Yes. Well, I'm very sorry to debrief this way, but Matt shouldn't have shown you this patient. I wanted to prepare you. It's been a shock to all of us.' The smile fades as quickly as it formed. He taps his keyboard and stares at the screen. 'Amitriptyline overdose. Not enough to kill him outright, but enough to make sure he ends up downstairs with nephrotoxicity and liver enzymes off the charts. And you're sure nothing about him rings a bell?'

'Doctor Morris, you know my...' I trail off. How do I find a convenient phrase for a lost childhood? '... you know my problems. I can't tell you things I don't know. It's as if you want me to pull a name out of thin air.'

The light from the screen reflects on his glasses as he turns towards me, obscuring his eyes and making him seem soulless, robotic.

'Okay. Is there anything else you'd like to add?'

I shake my head. *No.* I just want to start the shift again as though this patient had never arrived.

'We'll leave it there then. I suppose it won't affect his treatment whether you know his identity or not. It'll be a miracle if we can keep him alive long enough for you to ever find out though,' Morris mutters, glancing at the toxicology results on the screen. 'I'll be sending you home today, of course.'

'Why?'

'Well, I'd have thought that'd be obvious?'

'No, really. I'll be okay.'

'Doctor Carter, I don't want you involved in his care.'

All I can hear in his condescending tone and clipped accent is that I'm fragile. A brittle young neurotic who needs protecting from myself, from my own past. Deep breaths, Edie.

'I want to stay at work today. My skills in ICU—'

'This is nothing to do with your skills.'

'So what is it about? My memory of this man?' I hesitate. 'Or lack thereof?'

'No. It's about my duty of care to you.'

He stands and walks to the window, staring down towards the ambulances queueing outside the Emergency Department at the far end of the building. A siren fades into the clear, washed-out May sky, whooping and warbling, as one slaloms its way into the distance. The places I can't – or won't – go to in my mind, the dead ends, make him uncomfortable. *I* make him uncomfortable. I'm a problem he can't fix, and it sometimes feels like it has become an obsession with him.

'Doctor Morris, can I ask you something?'

'Go ahead.'

'Why was my agreeing to cognitive therapy a condition of you taking me on?'

He turns, his pale eyes steady behind his wire-framed glasses. His emotions always live and die in an instant, flicking across his features like a spark in the breeze. Was there a moment of genuine compassion? Something beneath the façade for once?

'Repression is never healthy. I'm thinking about your welfare, so is Doctor Wilson.'

'So the fact I desperately needed this placement didn't come into it?'

'No. Therapy is for your benefit, not mine. Self-awareness makes you a better doctor.'

'I'm already a good doctor.'

'I know. So accept our help.'

More than ever, I feel like one of Morris's patients, a specimen for examination and classification. The way he tries to read my mind feels like an invasion. Worse still is the way he and Wilson wilfully misunderstand how it feels, as if I enjoy being this way. As if I'm failing to grasp my own condition, blissfully aware of my own imperfections.

'I don't need protecting from this patient,' I tell him. 'I want to be involved.'

'Edie, I'm sorry for the shock you've had. But in this situation, you don't get to choose.' Morris returns to his seat and adopts the same position, fingertips supporting his chin. 'If you insist on remaining at work, then I'm putting you on the urology list while this man is with us. You will stay out of the ICU.'

'And if I don't?'

'Why are you so intent on defying me?'

'Doctor Morris, just because I don't remember who he is doesn't mean I can't be involved in his care.'

'I'm afraid it does,' he replies quietly.

'And if I refuse?'

He sighs. 'If you choose to directly ignore my decision, you may jeopardise your progression at this hospital.'

So he's using my career as a weapon? As he gazes implacably towards the window, I revise my attitude towards him. He's more than difficult, he's impossible. Condescending, infuriating, take your pick. If there was a flicker of anything other than authoritarian aloofness in his expression, it has long gone. I don't win conversations like this with Morris, but I do get to fight another day.

'What about the police?' I ask as I stand to leave, imagining difficult interviews with stony-faced officers, as they sit and write notes with cynical expressions. Judging me, probing. It's hard enough talking to Morris and Wilson about the past, never mind complete strangers.

Morris drifts back into the room from some distant place. Without replying, he uncoils from his chair, tall and thin. Silently, he holds the door open for me, the meeting over. The noises of the hospital filter along the corridor. A trolley clanging, distant talking, a lift pinging.

I hesitate. 'Doctor Morris, the police? Have you checked with them?'

He frowns briefly. I wait for an answer, which is forever in coming.

'No,' he replies. 'I want to keep this whole thing in-house. We don't need a circus.'

He flashes a terse smile as he ushers me out, but for once the gaze from his frost-blue eyes does not hold mine. The door clicks shut, leaving me alone in the empty corridor, as I begin to understand what the look on his face meant. I've been here for two years and never seen anything other than absolute certainty on his thin features. But he'd let the mask slip and, by the time it was back on, I'd noticed. His perfect, balanced world has wobbled on its axis, just like mine. Perhaps we're not so different after all, Doctor Morris.

I saw it in your eyes.

You're as scared of this patient as I am.

5

Edie

Harry could quote chapter and verse on why fear equals fascination, and why we do the very things we know we shouldn't. Excessive activity in the amygdala, dopamine overload, adrenaline fix. Any number of psychological reasons why I've taken less than an hour to break Morris's rule. As soon as Morris was in a meeting, I'd crept back to the patient's bedside and closed the curtains behind me. For the last five minutes, I've been watching the scarred chest rise and fall in time with the ventilator. My eyes have followed each crease of his forehead, every contour of his chin and angle of his face, waiting for a flash of recognition, a glimpse of something I can grab hold of and drag into the light.

Nothing.

I let my fingers touch his cheek, brush his closed eyes. Behind the jaundiced lids, what have they seen? What do they remember? If I leaned across now, and gazed into them, what would they tell me? My hand hovers, uncertain. Perhaps the saying is true; the eyes contain the soul. My arm drops to my side.

I'm not ready to look, and I'm not sure I ever will be.

I quickly scan his notes. Most of his patient record is either blank or invented. First name: *Unknown*. Surname: *Male*. Date of birth: *1 January 1970 (estimated)*. Address, *NFA*, allergies, *unknown*. With one eye on the door to the unit, I scroll through Morris's admission notes and scan the treatment plan. That pompous git is right about one thing, the blood results are appalling. I flick back, scrolling again, frowning. I read his history, or what there is of it. Multiple old scars, query cause. New wounds across the chest. At this, my pulse races as the jagged words *forgive me* form in my mind again. Found unconscious outside the Emergency Department having already overdosed. Amitriptyline bottles in his jacket. No identification or birthmarks. Nothing that gives away anything about his past.

Except his message to me.

Morris will be livid if he sees how quickly I've ignored his instructions, so I slink back across the unit. I've almost made it to the link corridor when in my peripheral vision a female nurse spots me and homes in. It's Jaz, thank God; slight and bird-like, with a dark ponytail that bounces against her oversized scrubs as she hurries towards me. I'm so relieved I could hug her. I don't have to; she hugs me first. Concern and curiosity combine in her dark eyes, and her usually expressive face is tight with a frown as we separate. Jaz can be a complex mix of extreme moods and contradictions; I have sometimes wondered how she makes such a good ICU nurse. She is often animated, impulsive, buzzing with energy. Yet a sudden, impenetrable layer of calm always envelops her when an emergency arises, a cool efficiency that spreads to the whole team. Right now, all of these things are bubbling under at once.

'What did he say to you, Edie?'

'Who?' I try to keep my voice steady.

'Don't give me that. *Morris*. You look like you're trying to smuggle the crown jewels out under your scrubs, honey. Everyone in the department is talking about what's happened.'

Inside, I groan. The last thing I want is to be the latest conversation piece in the unit. It's not even ten o'clock and I'm already drained, with the spectre of Amy Wilson's therapy session still hovering over me. I don't even want to think about the dinner party. My phone has pinged at least six times this morning with Harry's texts.

It doesn't matter if you're late, Edes. Just come along.

Left unanswered, they'd finally tailed off, tersely.

Okay, I get the message.

Ignoring him is a cowardly way of ducking out, but he'll understand when he knows what's happened.

'Well?' Jaz probes.

'He said I'm not to have anything to do with our man in there.' I glance back towards the bay. 'So I'm in theatres for a while. The urology list.'

'Eurrgh. Ten hours a day of octogenarian genitals.' She grimaces, pulling me aside. 'So if you're supposed to stay away from our mystery psychopath, why did I see you coming out of his cubicle?'

'Doesn't anything get past you?'

She rolls her eyes. *Dumb question.*

Jaz is one of those people I can't hide from. In two years, we've already shared too much about ourselves for any walls to remain. As she looks at me, something in our eyes connects, and I can feel my composure slipping. When I landed on the wards as a third-year student and things got real, I'd always found somewhere private to press the release valve, ducking into the nearest sluice room, drug cupboard or linen store to vent my feelings alone. Never let it show, I promised myself, and until I'd met Jaz I'd been true to my word. Now, as tears sting my eyes, I clench my jaw so hard my teeth hurt. At least it's Jaz who is seeing me unguarded, even for a moment. Her face softens.

'Hey, I'm sorry, hon.' She strokes my arm. 'Are you okay?'

'Yeah.'

She studies my face for a moment, then pulls me towards the drug cupboard, our ad-hoc meeting room. Inside, we're so close it's even harder to hide my feelings.

'Edie, it's me you're talking to.'

'No, I'm fine.' I shake my head and my gaze drops from hers.

Then she is reaching out to me, holding me, as the last fragment of my resolve finally gives way and I'm crying on her shoulder, my tears darkening the fabric of her light navy scrubs to midnight blue. She holds me in silence, as I let the shock and fear of seeing this patient come rolling out. Through the tears I can see that she has put her foot against the door, so no one can come in and see me like this. It's a small instinctive action on her part, but one I appreciate more than she probably realises. She knows how I would feel if anyone else saw me this emotional; she understands me better than almost anyone in my life except Harry, and it's all there in that protective gesture. After dozens of heart-to-heart talks over bottles of wine, she knows my confidence rests on a very fragile image of myself.

Finally, I lift my head, and rub my eyes. 'It's been a crazy day, you know? I don't know what to do.' I push a long breath through pursed lips, forcing my work face back on.

'You go home. That's what you do.'

'No, Jaz, don't you see? Whoever this man is, I want to be part of his care. I'm not sure why, but I just do.'

'He's obviously unhinged, though, Edie. Damaged. You don't know what he's done.'

'Yeah, I know.'

'Matt is such a fucking idiot.' Jaz rips a square of blue tissue from the roll next to the door and dabs my eyes gently before handing it to me. 'I wish he'd never shown him to you like that this morning,' she says. 'It was thoughtless. Morris was not impressed with him.'

'Well, I'm glad he did. Honestly.'

'I should have been there to stop him.' She shakes her head. 'I don't know why you came back to the department, Edie. It's like you're torturing yourself. Why not be kind to yourself for once? You've told me before how it feels to have these gaps in your memory, how out of control you feel sometimes. When we first talked – you know, I mean really opened up to each other – I saw how you struggled to even speak about it.'

'So I keep running away from it?'

'It's not running away. It's coping. Just like I've moved on from my past. God knows I needed to. Whatever happened back then is over, Edie. We've talked about this. It's *now* that matters, not then.'

'I know, and that's why it makes more sense for me to carry on, Jaz. To keep involved. If not, I feel like I'm handing over even more control to my past.'

'And more control to Morris?' she says, perceptive as ever.

'Yes, that too, and he already treats me like he owns me.'

She snorts angrily. 'Morris is such a dick. Be careful, Edie, he hates being defied. If he sees you here, he'll find a way of paying you back.'

I manage a short, sour laugh. 'He already has. Therapy sessions with Amy Wilson.'

'Come!'

Amy Wilson's muffled voice filters through the thick, heavily panelled oak door of her office. Inside, she is tidying the books that line the walls. Small and busy, she has to stand on tiptoe to reach the middle shelves. Her neatly bobbed, dyed blonde hair has rogue streaks of grey showing at the roots, and her glasses have slid halfway down her sharp nose. She peers at me over them.

'Ahhh, Edie. Come in. Sit down.'

I sit, already checking the time. I don't make a good patient, doctors never do. Wilson adjusts her glasses and sits opposite, sipping from a cup of liquid that smells like stewed dandelions.

'Can I get you some tea?'

The shake of my head is probably too emphatic. 'No, thanks.'

'So how are you? Am I going to meet resistance again this week?'

'I don't think I've been particularly resistant.'

We both recognise the lie, but to her credit, she simply nods and re-adjusts her glasses. 'No, maybe resistance was the wrong word. Are you going to finally buy into these sessions, though?'

'I'll try.'

'Excellent. It's important, now more than ever, that you understand the mechanics of your dissociation.'

'What do you mean, now more than ever?'

'Well, given what happened today,' she says. 'The mystery patient?'

I straighten in my chair. 'Have you been talking to Doctor Morris?'

'Of course. We talk all the time.'

The fact I'm being discussed behind my back settles into my stomach like a lump of granite. I force a bitter smile, feeling like a schoolgirl caught smoking behind the science block. 'Well, you can relax,

Amy. Doctor Morris has made sure I won't be involved in the case.'

'Good. Dissociative amnesia like yours always has a definite pathology, Edie. The way to access these traumatic events safely, and I emphasise the word safely, is in a controlled way. We discover things slowly, not…' she pauses, handling the words daintily '… through sudden shocks like this.'

'I'm really not that delicate, Amy,' I lie, remembering the drug cupboard this morning.

'Hmmm.' Wilson drags my file towards her from the corner of the desk, opens it, and scans briefly. She is old-school; despite the computer on her desk, she writes copious notes on a yellow legal pad as we talk. I've grown to hate that fucking pad. She looks up and adjusts her glasses again. 'You know, it's interesting how trauma works. Sometimes we repress things that have been done to us; other times we repress things we have done to others.' I wait for her to continue, although I know where this is going; *it's your fault, Edie. You're the only one who can access the truth.* 'Either way, outside of physical causes, true amnesia is something of a myth. Research is making this clearer to us now. What you have is an inability to recall certain events, that's all. It's all in there, Edie, we just need to tease it out. We need to get used to that idea.'

'*We* need to get used to it, do we?'

'There's that barrier again, Edie.'

My hackles rise at her measured, analytical gaze. 'Do you think I enjoy being this way, Doctor Wilson? Incomplete? As if it's some kind of game to me?'

'No, of course not. But we need to understand the context of the repressive drive, which means you need to engage with me.' She sips her drink. 'For example, in previous sessions we have identified certain landmarks in your failure to recall. The death of your father when you were eight, for instance, is a lost memory. Equally, we have established an approximate age when your memories become more lucid. One particularly significant event was at twelve, when you moved towns and started at your new school.'

Yes, that memory is crystal clear. A fresh September morning, seventeen years ago. I can still hear the forced optimism of my mother. *New town, new school, Edie.* Her tone of bright, precarious confidence. *A new start, my love, for both of us. This house has too many memories.*

Ever since I sat down at Wilson's desk, my forefinger has been rubbing impulsively against the quick of my thumb, picking it roughly; a teenage habit I hadn't succumbed to for ages. Now, as I think of that year, a sharp pain shoots through my hand as the skin tears. I suck the blood away as Wilson continues, blithely checking notes.

'Oak Green, wasn't it?' she asks.

My heart trips faster, the name of the school jarring as it leaves her lips. I can't hide my shock, and she leans forward. She notices the blood on my thumb.

'Are you okay, Edie? Can I get you a plaster?'

'No, I'm fine.'

'I've never categorised your changing schools as a traumatic memory. Were you unhappy there?'

'Yes. But no more than most.'

'So why the reaction when I mentioned the name of the school?' She closes the file and pushes it away, sipping her tea.

'Because I've never told you it.'

Her composure slips. 'But you must have.'

Now it's my turn to lean forward, elbows on the desk. 'Doctor Wilson, I've never told you the name of my secondary school. So why is it in your notes?'

'Edie. Look, we have your best interests at heart. Trust me.'

'So I keep being told.' I stand and zip my hoodie, then sling my bag over my shoulder dismissively. 'Sorry, I'm done for today.'

Wilson stands too, her lips tight, eyes flinty. 'You need to address this trauma, Edie. You need to face the past.'

'Maybe. But on my terms. Not yours.'

Her frustrated stare burns the back of my neck all the way to the door. Outside, in the oak-panelled corridor, which smells of floor polish and ancient pipe smoke, I lean against the wall and take deep breaths.

Wilson and Morris can make me attend these sessions until they both retire, but I'm never going to share with either of them those things which I do remember. Those splintered pieces, still jagged and painful after all these years, which take me unaware and are just as quickly suppressed, leaving me feeling as though I'm treading deep water over some dark abyss where vague, nameless shadows are slithering below.

There is a large sash window at the end of the corridor, showing a corner of the new wing where the ICU is. I can sense his presence there. Much as I want to wish him away, he's here.

I check my phone. Six-thirty. I've kept it together today, against all the odds. But right now, I need a drink, and I'm not drinking on my own. Even a dinner party at the Creightons' is better than being left alone with my thoughts.

6

Harry

My phone pings. Edie.

I'll be there in about half an hour. I've just called the taxi.

Heart pounding, I glance across the kitchen to where Nicky is chatting to my mother. After Edie had ignored my messages, I was certain she wouldn't be coming. I quickly tap a reply.

Don't bother, they've invited my ex.

My thumb hovers on send. Why should it be Edie who has to stay at home? Who cares if Nicky is here, anyway? Let everyone see Edie and me together; it'll be a statement, make it clear how we feel about each other. Nicky might be a friend of the family, but my parents knew exactly what they were doing when they invited her. So why give them the satisfaction?

I delete the message and fire off another.

Can't wait to see you.

As far as Edie is concerned, my parents disliked her from the start, thought that she wasn't good enough. I don't believe it was quite that simple, but I understand her logic. Edie has experienced their judgemental traits in small doses; I've lived with them. From the moment I arrived at the sprawling house in Willenhall Lane an hour ago, the claustrophobia of my childhood began seeping into my psyche as if by osmosis. My mother and father were the original helicopter parents, they wrote the book. Nothing I ever did was unwatched, unmeasured or unassessed for its value in my development. Everything had a purpose in the parental project, and I still feel like a child again whenever I come back to the family home. Regression, the classic stress response. No wonder I went a little overboard as a student when I got to Cambridge. I had a lot of freedom to catch up on.

I listen for the doorbell, getting steadily more uptight. It's important that my parents realise this relationship is for real. Edie and I have been engaged for well over a year, so why isn't that enough to convince them? Why can't they just let her be herself, comfortable in her own skin, allowing her to be whoever she needs to be? Instead, they constantly try to make her just like them or, worse still, a clone of Nicky. Even when I explained that Edie had a difficult childhood, they never thawed. They just saw someone withdrawn, impenetrable. But I got used to her being that way, falling in love with her by instalments as she let fragments of herself emerge, allowing me into her life, sharing her secrets. Her father's death, her mother's depression. We'd been together for eighteen months when she sat me down one night and, over several bottles of wine and frequent tears, told me that nearly everything she knew about her early childhood was second-hand information, drip fed by her mother and sewn together like a quilt with half the patches missing.

She didn't need to tell me what dissociation was, I'd seen it before. Our link to the past isn't as solid as we think it is, and all our memories are fictions really, just stories we write about ourselves. In some cases, when the story is unbearable enough, people just tear the pages out completely as Edie had done. She and her mother had settled into their routine and had found a compromise, and Edie had asked me to do the same. I'd readily promised. Accept me for the person I am now, Edie said. If my mother and I can get by without raking up our past, you and I can too. And I've always kept my promise because it was in that moment of vulnerability that I first knew I loved her. My parents have never seen her like that; open, emotionally raw, baring her soul. The simple fact is, they don't know Edie the way I do.

As I'm getting another drink, the doorbell chimes, sending my pulse racing again. Talking constantly, my mother shows Edie into the kitchen. Edie looks stunning in a black cocktail dress, her dark hair piled in a loose updo and her kohl-rimmed eyes almost jade in the kitchen downlights. Her expression says she's being made to feel like she's performed the worst social gaffe in history by arriving last. My father watches her slyly, as he holds court by the new kitchen range with a few smartly dressed management types from the Royal College of Psychiatrists who have travelled up from London. Gathering them in that spot was no accident. The range is a La Cornue and, although he is not vulgar enough to tell them outright how much it cost, he never misses the chance to make a non-verbal statement. I've been hovering on the periphery, half-listening to him talk about government select committees, strategic planning, and some new clinical directorship role he has secured at some private facility. Private care, just another one of the many pies he likes to have his fingers planted firmly in. He sure knows how to follow the money.

As though caught in the middle of some conspiracy, he immediately stops talking shop as Edie approaches and treats her to an interrogative smile. 'Edie. Glad you could make it. How's anaesthetics? Still putting people to sleep?'

Edie stiffens and I step in quickly. 'Not as effectively as your conversations do, Dad. Excuse us a moment.' I guide her towards the drinks, grab the bottle of Rioja I've already half-finished and pour us both half a glass. As Edie drinks some I swallow mine in one go, ignoring the sidelong frown from my father. In a moment of frustration, I bang the empty glass down on the marble loud enough to make people nearby look across. 'Why does he have to be such a sanctimonious prick?'

'Harry, calm down.' Edie glances around her nervously as people go back to their conversations.

'Yeah.' I top us both up, and clink her glass with an apologetic smile. 'Forget him. Are you okay?'

'Yeah, I guess.'

'Thanks for coming. I really wanted you to be here.' I stand facing the room so she can't see Nicky yet. 'Edes, listen. I've got something to confess. Don't get mad, but—'

'Actually, I'm not okay, Harry,' she interrupts, her mind elsewhere.

36

'Something's happened. Can we find somewhere quiet to talk for a while?'

'Yeah, of course. But I need to explain something first.'

Her arrival announced by a waft of lavender perfume, my mother manoeuvres herself between us, her hostess grin fixed. 'Now then, Harry, don't let Edie be antisocial as usual. She needs to meet the gang.'

Edie throws me a glance. *Please get me out of this.*

But I'm too slow. Her hand slips from mine, and she is steered around the party to my mother's running commentary. *This is Godfrey, he's something in the City. Meet Madeleine, she runs a small gallery in Frith Street.*

She is moved on continuously. Circulated, like a strange exhibit. Meanwhile, I'm frozen, watching the slow-motion car crash about to happen. My mother turns her one last time, and then Edie is face to face with Nicky.

They are the same age, but Nicky is a couple of inches taller. She tosses her brown curls and shows her straight, white teeth, holding out her hand as my mother introduces them.

No one notices the confusion behind Edie's polite, rictus smile.

But I do, and I immediately wish I'd sent that first text instead.

'Harry, what the fuck were they thinking, inviting your ex?'

Her words break ten minutes of icy silence. To his credit, ever since picking us up, the taxi driver has appeared oblivious to the strained atmosphere in the back of his cab.

'I'm sorry, Edes, honestly. I was trying to tell you before you saw her. It's not like I invited her myself.'

'You could have told me in advance.'

'I didn't want her there. She's just a friend of the family.'

'She's a moron.' She takes a deep, ragged breath. 'She still wants you, you know.'

'Well, who wouldn't?' I immediately regret the attempt to lighten the mood.

'Life's one big bloody joke to you, isn't it?'

'Okay, if you want the truth, I wanted Nicky to see us together. Just like I want you and my parents to get on, however unlikely that now seems. We're engaged, Edie. I love you, not her. I don't know if my mother even thought about—'

'Oh, she thought about it all right. They both did.'

In the strobing flashes of the passing streetlights, Edie's green eyes fizz with anger. Rain has begun falling lightly on the windows, and the driver, still pretending to be deaf, flicks his wipers on.

'Okay,' I say. 'But why should you have to avoid her? It's you I love.'

'You barely said a word to me all night. What kind of love is that?'

'Everyone was talking at once. It was a dinner party.'

'Harry, I've somehow kept things together today, and now this. You knew I wanted some time with you, that I had something on my mind.' She turns away, staring at the road as it hisses by. 'It's been a hard day.'

'So talk now then, if that's what you want.'

She leans towards the driver, her expression impenetrable. 'Stop here, please.'

'Edes, wait.'

The driver checks in the rear-view mirror. Noticing that he is looking to me for confirmation, Edie leans closer. 'You don't need his bloody permission. Stop the car.'

He pulls to the kerb. In the mirror, his eyes find mine with a clear message. *I don't need this shit, mate.* Edie pulls the door open.

'Edie, what are you doing? We're a mile from home.'

'I'll walk. I need some air.'

And then she's out and striding along the deserted Harborne street, pulling the hood of her coat up. I fish some notes out of my pocket and thrust them into the driver's hand. I have no idea how much I've given him. 'Stay here for a minute, would you?'

I sprint to catch up with her. I grab her shoulders and turn her towards me. Her cheeks are wet with more than the rain, and she is shaking.

'I'm sorry, Ede. Honestly. I'm stupid, I'm clumsy. I didn't mean to hurt you.' I wrestle with the words to put things right. 'I wanted to make a statement to them all. About us.'

She holds herself, pulling herself inwards. Why didn't I see what an ordeal it had been? Edie had spent half the evening listening to Nicky bragging about her new junior partnership in some Silver Circle law firm, all the while glancing maliciously across the table towards us. She had always had that bitchy element, ever since we dated at university.

According to Edie, first love always lingers, but she's wrong.

'Look, it's not anything you've done,' she whispers, so quietly I can hardly hear above the hiss of the rain. 'It's something else.'

'So what's the matter then? Please.'

The words catch for a moment, jamming in her throat. 'Harry, he's found me.'

She is breathing hard now, her eyes wide with the fear of someone drowning, going under. We are alone in the street, and the taxi has driven off. A bedroom light goes on in the terraced house next to us, the curtain twitching. Hating my dutiful, deep-rooted sense of propriety, I guide Edie further along the street, my arm around her shoulders. At the corner, I wait as her breathing slows.

'Who's found you?'

'I don't know.'

'You're not making any sense, Edes.'

Gradually, choosing her sentences like someone feeling their way along a tightrope, she tells me about the unidentified patient. About his wounds, the message. Morris. About Wilson digging into her past. As she talks, she becomes more focused, more in control. As the full ordeal of her day unfolds, I take her hand, fumbling around in vain for something to say. Working out what people need to hear comes naturally to me in clinical settings, but here, when it counts, I'm mute. Finally, I fall back on that time-honoured platitude that men use when we've run out of options.

'Don't worry. It'll be okay.'

She shakes her head. Her voice is quiet, weary. 'Why is he here? Why now? I'd found a balance in my life, and now this.'

'Look, whatever he's done, this man can't harm you any more. Take some time off work. Don't give him any more power over you.'

'No, you don't get it.'

'What do you mean?'

'Harry, I'm not running any more. I'm going to find out what happened, who he is.' I can feel the tension in her fingers laced through mine. 'That's why I'm frightened.' A fear is growing in me too, taking root. But what choice do I have?

'I'll help you, Edes. We'll do it together. Okay?'

She reaches up and touches my cheek. I kiss her, and she responds. Our kiss feels the same as it always has. When I snake my arms around her waist, it feels the same. It's this beautiful, hard-won familiarity that feeds the fear.

Edie has buried the past for a reason. And if she uncovers it, I'm scared that everything is going to change.

7

Edie

I stare into the darkness at five-thirty and my arm stretches out across Harry's side of the bed. It must have been empty for some time because nothing remains of him there, no indentation or warmth on the sheets. My eyes are burning like I've come off the wrong end of a long night shift, but I must have dozed at some point, because I dreamed of a cubicle in a silent, empty ICU. A low-lit department, all the beds vacant except for one. The man was lying there, but this time young and healthy. No endotracheal tube in his mouth, no central line in his jugular vein, no infusions pumps, no monitors recording his body's slow decline. He had no scarring, no cuts, no jaundice. He was resting as if asleep and, as I watched him, his eyes opened. Green eyes, lighter than mine. Then he smiled in wordless recognition.

As the dream fades, my thoughts drift to the overwhelming need to run away, which had blindsided me in the taxi last night. I have a mantra that has followed me throughout my life, instilled by the blind faith of my mother. *We'll cope.* I internalised it, repeated it, made it my own. It got me through school, university, medical training; gave me an edge of defiance. It was my mother's favourite phrase during my teenage years, long before she ignored her own advice and spectacularly stopped coping. Years of medication, institutions and therapy have separated us, but still I cope, like a loyal daughter. But what would happen if I ever followed her down that dark path? What happens when something gets through the armour? Last night happens, I guess.

Downstairs, the smell of coffee hits me as I enter the kitchen. I'm not rushing for once; the clock reads quarter to six. Harry is at

41

the breakfast bar in a sloppy jumper and checked pyjama bottoms. A stray lock of hair flops across his forehead, above eyes that are as sleep deprived as mine. As I come in, concern deepens the lines on his face.

'How are you feeling?' he asks.

'I'm okay. I'm sorry about last night.'

'Not as sorry as me.' He stands up and hugs me. He has been sitting close to the heavy iron radiator and his body heat encloses me. I shut my eyes briefly, sinking into the warmth. He rubs my back and kisses the top of my head. 'I shouldn't have made last night all about me and my parents.'

Head on his chest, I let myself be held. After we arrived home soaked through, Harry and I had showered, gone to bed and talked into the small hours. I'd told him everything again, with no detail or emotion left out; the patient, the words on his skin, the feeling my whole fractured life had telescoped into a single moment, too intense to bear. I believed Harry when he whispered that the past can't hurt me; it sounded true coming from him. His hand found mine as I talked, stroking it, and afterwards we'd made love, everything else forgotten for a while.

'Stay at home,' he continues. 'Let other people deal with it today.'

I head towards the coffee machine and pour myself a cup, spooning two sugars in. I'm going to need caffeine and carbs more than ever today. I swallow some immediately, enjoying the mild burning sensation sinking through my chest. 'And then do what? Brood on it?'

'Edie, you always keep things in until it's too late, like last night. Give yourself a break for once.'

'Last night was a one-off. When have you ever seen me like that before?'

'Never. But that proves my point. If I was your doctor, I would insist you stay off work for a few days.'

'Good job you're not my doctor then. I'm not some fragile little flower. Storming out of the taxi last night was embarrassing.'

He gets up and pours himself another cup, shaking his head. 'Embarrassing? It was a clinical manifestation of stress, Edes.' He gives me that *I'm meeting you halfway* expression. 'I realise the Nicky thing didn't help, and I know Dad is hard work sometimes, but even so. Outbursts of emotion? Paranoia?' He wipes away the bead of fresh blood on my thumb where I've been picking at it. 'Compulsive tics? Do you want a proper diagnosis, Doctor Carter?'

'No. I want a shower.' I kiss his cheek and slip back out into the cool of the hallway before he can answer.

The main cafeteria at the KG is in a wide rotunda, with a high glass ceiling and tall windows. Flooded with light, it echoes with the clacking of cutlery and crockery, cutting through the buzz of conversation from patients and relatives, nurses and doctors, all mixing together in a nebulous, noisy lunchtime crowd. I spot Jaz stretched out on one of the central sofas, wearing a cardigan over blue scrubs, her right leg folded over the left in a half-lotus position. I queue for two coffees and then wander over. She straightens and grins.

'Trust you to be late, Doctor Carter. How's the urology list?'

'Too graphic by far. It's putting me off sex for life,' I say with a shrug. She snorts laughter as I hand her a coffee. 'And some of those urology surgeons are complete throwbacks. It's like being stuck in the locker room of a public school rugby team.'

'Be grateful you didn't get orthopaedics. Those guys make the Bullingdon Club seem enlightened.' She notices the dark rings under my eyes. 'Hey, you look terrible.'

'Thanks.' The sarcasm falls flat. 'I didn't sleep well, not surprisingly. Come on then, don't keep me waiting. What's been going on?'

'Okay. Our man… no improvement yet. Morris is keeping this guy very much to himself; he doesn't like us doing anything without supervision. He's all over this case like a rash.'

'I can imagine. I've also discovered Wilson has been checking up on my past herself, and you know how tight her and Morris are. I bet they're filling in the gaps themselves.'

'Are you serious? They've got no right. For God's sake, Edie, we all have things we'd like to bury deep enough to forget.' Her brow furrows, a shadow of pain. 'You know what I mean.'

I nod; Jaz pays for her extreme emotions with extreme self-analysis, and she often finds herself lacking. As I do. Perhaps we bonded so quickly when we first started working together because of it. Harry or Amy Wilson might call it trauma bonding, but that's too dismissive a word for a complicated connection. There have been times when I have woken in the night to the light of my phone buzzing. A call for help from Jaz, when she has let her darker thoughts get the better of her. I've seen the Citalopram in her bathroom cabinet. The faded lateral scars across her upper arm, careful and methodical signs of teenage self-loathing, now hidden to the rest of the world beneath the t-shirt and scrubs. Yes, I know exactly what Jaz means when she talks about burying her past.

'Why are we both so fucked up?' I take her hand.

'All the most interesting people are.' She smiles, and the introspection fades. 'Your past is no more relevant to your competence than mine. Wilson is out of order.'

The acrid aftertaste of Wilson's deception, as the name of my old school slipped so casually out of her mouth, still lingers. 'Yeah. Trust me, she knows things about me that I haven't shared with her yet.'

'Shit, talk about unethical.' She pauses, studying me over the rim of her cup. 'Listen, do you really want to know who this guy is?'

I shrug, staring at my coffee. Until yesterday, everything was going so smoothly. I was happy to exist in ignorance. Okay, not blissful ignorance, but at least a version of it. I could have played along with Wilson and Morris until I qualified as an anaesthetist. Maybe I still can. Then in a few months I could move to a different hospital, a few years after that make consultant. Then what? Marriage, kids, big house? School PTA and village fete committees? The whole clichéd picture of happiness, which deep down I would probably hate. But at least I would be normal, and those vague shadows from my childhood wouldn't matter any more.

'To be honest, Jaz, until yesterday's session with Wilson, I would have said no. But I need to know what *they* know. Wilson, Morris. I don't want to be treated like a freak show exhibit any more.'

'Where was the guy found again?'

'Outside the emergency entrance.'

Jaz's dark eyes flash with inspiration. Excited, she grabs my elbow, clattering my cup and saucer. Two elderly people at the next table glare at us. 'Well, don't you see?' She searches my face. 'CCTV? He'll have been filmed arriving.'

I hold her gaze, shaking my head in disbelief. CCTV, why didn't I think of that? 'Jaz, you're a genius. Perhaps he came with someone. Maybe he had a car, took a taxi?'

'Always trust a nurse to think laterally.' Jaz grins. 'Well, drink up then. You know where the security guys live, Edie. They'll have seen him coming in.'

I give myself one last chance to escape the decision. I'm existing on adrenaline, and the past is rushing at me too fast, screaming to be heard. It's one thing to see him lying immobile on an ICU bed. But to see him on screen, walking, moving. To watch his body language. It's becoming too real. 'I don't know, Jaz.'

She doesn't hesitate. 'Yes you do, Edie. This might be against my better judgement, but what are friends for but to support each other? You said you want to know, and it's the truth. I can see it in your eyes.' She stands, encouraging me to do the same. 'And there's no time like the present.'

8

Edie

In a street on the border of Ladywood and Winson Green, the daylight is fading across a row of dilapidated Victorian houses. Only a few hours ago, I was in the security team's Portakabin, watching a monitor as people scuttled in and out of the hospital in fast-forward. Beside me at the desk Jamie, a lanky thirty-year-old in a poorly fitting black bomber jacket and cargo pants, swivelled a joystick like a seasoned gaming addict as he sped through the footage. He'd swallowed my story about needing to trace a patient's medical background with a nonchalant grunt.

The unknown patient had been found just before seven in the evening. As Jamie searched the video, ambulances flew in and whizzed away, their blue lights a blur. Cars slipped rapidly in and out of parking spaces. Towards six-fifteen the speed of the footage gradually slowed. Then a taxi pulled up near the entrance and a man got out.

It was unmistakably him. Tall, perhaps six foot one, staggering slightly. That made sense; toxicology showed elevated alcohol levels. As I watched him, my chest tightened. It was the way he walked, the way his shoulders rolled. A ghostly remnant of something – somebody – familiar. He sat on a bench, took a small bottle of tablets out of his jacket, and began swallowing. His jacket was half-zipped, and I could make out the blood staining his t-shirt.

'Who are the taxi firm?' I asked. The footage had dragged me in, holding me there.

Jamie spooled back and squinted at the screen.

'Arrow. 343-7215.'

46

'I need to find his next of kin. Could you ring the company for me, find his address? It'd sound more official coming from security.'

Jamie grunted again, no longer interested in my reasons. 'I guess so.'

As he made the call, I phoned Harry. It rang out to voicemail.

'Harry? I'm really sorry but I'm going to be late getting home tonight. The list has dragged on. Sorry, I know you were planning to cook. Love you lots.'

I cut off, decision made. After watching this man come to find me, seeing him overdose, it was already too late to go back.

Now, in the grey light of dusk, the streetlight reveals the taxi firm's pickup address; a large, double-fronted house with dirty brickwork and broken guttering. In some of the grimy windows, blankets and sheets hang in place of curtains. An overgrown hedge obscures the front garden. Thanks to a six-month community placement, I can recognise an HMO at first glance. They're always the same; large old houses, boxed into as many tiny rooms as the landlord can manage before they dump the most vulnerable in society there like battery chickens. Anyone who has fallen through the gaps. Poorly managed schizophrenics, ex-convicts and drug addicts, the lost and forgotten, one step away from sleeping under cardboard. In this darkening street I feel very alone, and every rational part of my mind is telling me not to subject myself to a risk like this. But then rationality has been in short supply since yesterday morning.

A cloud rises from near the unkempt hedge where a slouching figure is sucking on a vape, silhouetted by the lights of the house. Before I can change my mind, I'm out of the car and walking across the road. My chest is pounding, my breath catches. I recognise my fight-or-flight response kicking in and try to control it. I'm on a busy residential street; what could happen? Unconvinced, I get my phone out and make sure the emergency call button is ready. I can smell the vape now, a sweet, fruity tang at the back of my throat. The man is watching me approach, a wry, curious smile on his lips. He is my age, broad-faced and stubbled, his hair shaved at the sides with a thick, dark nest on top. He takes a deep drag before he speaks.

'You probation?' White vapour carries his words out. His voice is deep and has an East London edge.

I clear my throat, attempting authority. 'No, I'm a doctor.'

'I should have known. Probation always come mob-handed, like the bailiffs.'

He laughs at his own joke and then loses interest in me and walks back towards the house. After a few seconds I follow him, several steps behind. He opens the cracked, peeling front door onto a run-down hallway with stairs leading upwards. The rickety banister is chipped gloss, a fire regulation notice curls from the wall.

Noticing I've followed, he leaves the door open. 'Anyone who's medical is normally here to take someone away to the nuthouse.' He waits inside for me to come in. I hesitate and he furrows his brow, comically hurt. 'I get it. You don't trust me.'

I shake my head. 'No, it's—'

'It's all right, I don't blame you. Look at this place.' He sighs. 'Okay, I'm Danny. I'm currently on eighty milligrams of methadone a day. I've done four years inside and I don't intend to go back. I can't fight my way out of a crisp packet, and I respect women. Do you trust me now?' At a small table in the hallway, he shuffles through a pile of letters, reading the addresses. He shakes his head. 'There's never anything for me.'

I take small steps into the musty, sweat-scented hallway. 'I'm Doctor Carter. I work in intensive care at the King George. We have a patient we need information on.'

'You're young for a doctor.'

'I've just aged well.' He smiles and I warm to him. 'Danny, we think the patient lives here. He's in his fifties, greying hair. About six foot one or two. He's a drinker.'

'That narrows it down.'

'He has lots of scars. You know, self-harm. Some old, some more recent.'

A frown crosses his face. 'Yeah, I know the bloke. Why do you want to know about him?'

'I need information on his medical background. He's in ICU, very sick.'

'Yeah, he's sick all right.' Danny's expression is stony, his jaw tight. 'Sick in the fucking head. With any luck, whatever he's got is fatal. His room is first floor.'

'Have you got a key?'

'You don't need one. The lock's been broken in. Let's just say he wasn't too popular around here.'

He walks up the stairs, letting a hollow-eyed young man pass, track marks snaking below the sleeves of his baggy t-shirt. On the landing, Danny pushes a flimsy door. The lock is splintered. As the door swings open, the smell of stale alcohol and body odour hits me. The room is three metres square. A small sink stands in the corner, filthy with years of grime. The mirror above is broken. An old duvet half-covers a single bed with a stained mattress. Cans and bottles litter the ancient carpet.

Scattered receipts and universal credit slips cover a rickety, Formica-lined desk near the window. I pick up a small address book and flick through it. Most of the pages are empty.

Danny curls his lip. 'He said his name was Karl. He arrived about a month ago, said he'd moved into the area to be near a friend. We even got drunk together once or twice. Then one of the other lads saw some of his post and we discovered his real name. Samuel Cox.'

The name jars, ricochets off my memory for an instant. Then I'm drowning in the bleakness of this place, and I want Danny to stop talking. I want to clamp his mouth shut, block this out. What do I do against the tidal wave coming at me? I can already hear its roar. I fight the urge to sprint from the house and get back in the car. Keep driving and never stop.

He continues, relentless. 'So figuring he was hiding something, we looked him up online. That's when we found out what he'd done to that little girl.'

The fine hairs are standing up on my arms. I hardly recognise my own voice.

'What little girl?'

'Edith something. They didn't give her last name.'

The humming of a car engine runs through some deep, subterranean layer of my mind. We are driving and I am watching this scene run in front of my eyes. A passenger in a flickering, silent film. The shape in the driver's seat is silhouetted, a man's bulk, his shoulders broad. *Him?* His outline remains fixed in my mind, like an afterimage burned on the retina. If I could hold the image long enough, he would turn and I would see him. But something inside me closes, a door slamming shut.

'What did he do?' The words tug at my throat.

'What did he do? Shit, you don't want to know. We read the old reports online about what he had confessed to doing. Taking her, abusing her. He even pleaded guilty, as if he was proud of it. Some of the guys here wanted to kill him; they would have done a lot worse than slap him around if they hadn't been on probation.' I'm dimly aware of flinching as Danny touches my arm, his eyes concerned. 'Are you okay, love?'

'I'm fine.' My thumb is slippery with blood, as my fingernail digs deeper and harder into the quick.

Danny takes his phone out. He taps, scrolls. 'Fucking nonce,' he growls. Then he shows me the screen, scrolling through the reports, pointing with a nail-bitten finger.

Samuel Cox. The man in my ICU. Younger, just like he was in my dream. Then I am looking through the glass of the phone screen at a carefree child smiling from the photo in a news report. She is impossibly small, barely recognisable.

'This is her?' I whisper, holding the screen towards him, not wanting to look any more.

'Yeah.' He looks at the picture, then at me. Does he see any similarity between the woman in front of him and the young girl in the picture? Do features really change as we grow older? He frowns as he glances between the screen and me but says nothing. I turn to the reports again, the words burning me.

Girl missing, eight.

Bile rises, my throat constricts.

Abducted.

The final word hits like the crash of waves on rocks.

Abused.

Then I'm in the corner and retching into the mould-stained sink.

9

Harry

The linguine carbonara has been congealing into a gloopy mess in the pan for two hours. How long can an elective theatre list go on for? I'm finishing my second glass of wine on an empty stomach and it's going to my head, shortening my patience. I drag my phone across the worktop, pause my playlist and thumb another text.

Edie, where are you? Dinner is looking like shit.

But I don't have time to press send, because as I'm typing the front door slams. I meet her in the hall as she throws her bag on the chair and sits on the stairs. A half-formed dig at how late she is dies on my lips. Her face is drawn and pale, and she frowns into thin air in that vacant, thousand-yard stare I've seen in catatonic patients. She doesn't meet my gaze.

'Edes, what's up?'

'I've just been driving around.' Her voice is flat, emotionless.

The linguine is forgotten. 'What's happened?'

She stares at the floor, frowning. 'I've spent the last hour driving aimlessly, and I can't recall a single moment of it.'

'What do you mean?' I ask. She is vague, unable to snap into the moment. 'Can I get you anything?'

'Harry, it's been right in front of me.'

'What has? Edie, you're freaking me out now.'

She looks at me for the first time since she came in. Her eyes are glassy with an emotion I can't place. Silently, she takes my hand and leads me to the kitchen. At the table, she pulls her laptop across and opens it. For several minutes she taps keys, searching with a concentration so intense I disappear.

Then she swivels the laptop towards me.

'Look.'

The browser is lined with tabs; she has opened a series of archived newspaper reports, laid out in old font, with none of the graphics and pop-up adverts most webpages have. Dated across two weeks in 2004 are reports, one after the other, giving lurid accounts of a child abduction. On every page there are details of a man called Samuel Cox, with long paragraphs speculating on his personal life and elaborate character portraits, painting a dramatic picture of a predator-in-waiting with unconcealed hysteria. I flick through the tabs. Cox in work suit and tie, quotes from colleagues and neighbours, a grainy picture of a young girl in her school uniform. Edie? Yes, I can see it now. The headlines come at me, in vivid, tabloid prose, straight from a summer twenty years ago. Edie's full name is not mentioned, but the press were having a field day regardless.

Seized in Somerset! Missing 8-Year-Old Girl Found in Coastal Village.

Cambridgeshire Man Charged with Kidnapping. Will Rot on Remand.

Throw Away the Key! Predator Samuel Cox Pleads Guilty Before Trial to Kidnapping and Sexual Abuse.

18 Years for Monster who Abducted and Abused Young Girl.

Edie is studying me, waiting for my response as I scroll through, my horror growing. It's him, the unknown patient. It has to be the thing she's been hiding from all this time and yes, she's right, it was all here for her to find if she'd wanted to. All it would have taken is some honesty from her mother and the will to look. But that's the whole point of dissociation, isn't it? There *is* no will to look. When it comes to trauma, more often than not ignorance is bliss.

A few years after her father died, she once told me, she and her mother moved away from their hometown, forcing themselves to look forward, not backward. With no close relatives, it was a clean start. It was their way of closing off the past physically as well as mentally. Now, beneath my empathy for them, a certainty is taking hold as I read the reports, confirming a suspicion I've had ever since Edie said Amy Wilson was researching her. Edie and her mother might not have had the will or the strength to face what happened to them, but others would have. It's human nature. But even if Morris and Wilson had searched her name online, finding what happened from that alone would have been almost impossible. Unlike the press, the police handled this carefully, sensitively. There was no huge public appeal, no naming the victim in full. A photograph of her had somehow slipped into one of the later reports, but otherwise the police had concentrated their efforts solely on finding the perpetrator. Efficiently going about their job. Tracking his car on motorway cameras, putting officers on the ground.

Whatever there was to be discovered about Edie, I'd always wanted it to come from her, and now it has. I once heard love described as an act of imagination, but it feels closer to an act of faith. Of believing in someone, no matter what. People like Jaz and me take Edie for who she is now, not her past. But there are plenty who won't. I move closer, wanting to hold her but feeling somehow clumsy, as if needing permission. She pulls the laptop towards her, flicking through the screens. I sit, waiting and watching. Occasionally she glances up at me, her fingernail grinding against her thumb, over and over. I take her hand, stopping her before she draws blood again.

I finally manage to say something. 'How did you find out?'

'There was CCTV at the hospital. I went to his bedsit, spoke to his neighbours.'

'Fuck. I mean… I can't—'

'It's all right, Harry. You don't have to find the words.'

I sigh. I'm supposed to be good at this. 'So what now?'

'I don't know.'

'What about talking to your mother about it?'

'No.' The force of her hand tearing from mine, and the hardening of her stare, is instant. I've seen some visceral responses to stress before, but the immediacy and power of her reaction resembles a lightning strike. Her hand hovers by her face, fingers splayed, before finally settling across her eyes as she rubs them wearily, the flash of tension dissipating. 'Harry, you know how unstable she can be. Are you suggesting I go rocking up to her house and shoving this in her face with no warning?'

'Well, you can't just brood on it. You have to either face it or forget it.'

'Thanks. For a psychiatrist you're pretty blunt. How many patients do you tell to just forget it?' Edie pushes herself upright, the tension in her neck and jaw muscles visible. She paces the kitchen, head in hands. Then, as if she's reached a tough decision, she pulls a small, battered address book from her pocket and drops it in front of me. 'I found this in his room.'

I flick through the book, mostly blank pages. There are only three entries. One is a taxi firm, the second is the probation service. The final number is written heavily, the pen scoring the paper. The name Melanie is scrawled above it. I shrug at Edie, and she taps the keyboard of the laptop and swivels it towards me again. On the screen there is a picture of a woman, dark-haired and slim, walking up the steps towards a Crown Court somewhere as she hurries from the cameras. I scan the caption.

Melanie Cox, thirty-four, wife of accused.

The woman in the photo must be in her fifties now. She will almost certainly have moved, doing exactly what Edie and her mother did by trying to put the whole thing behind her. The number in the address book will either be disconnected or invalid, or a complete stranger will answer. And even if she's still there, Melanie Cox will want nothing to do with Edie. Why would she? She will probably feel as guilty as Cox himself.

Edie is waiting, her hand resting on the address book. 'Well, what do you think?'

'Honestly? I don't know if this is the right thing.'

'You said you'd support me.'

Reluctantly, I nod. She'll do it whether I agree or not. Once she has decided on something, it's impossible to shift her. But I still find myself hoping that Melanie Cox has vanished from the face of the earth. Edie picks up the book and stares at me, waiting, her head tilted. *Well?*

'You want me to wait outside?'

'Yes, please.'

'Are you sure about doing this?'

'Harry, it's going to be hard enough without an audience.'

I kiss her and leave the room as she dials the number in Cox's phone book. I wait in the hall, nerves throbbing. The indecipherable, muffled hum of a one-sided conversation reaches me through the door. Her voice is low, a soft monotone. Then there is silence. When I go back in, Edie is standing at the sink, steaming water running.

I stroke her shoulder. 'Well?'

'She answered.'

'And?'

'She'll see me. But there was no shouting, no shock. I introduced myself and she sounded almost resigned. Like she had been expecting the call.'

'What else did she say?'

'That she has something to give me.'

Her tone is business-like, neutral. But as she runs her hands under the hot tap, the white enamel is running pink where her torn, bitten cuticle is oozing fat droplets of fresh blood.

10

Edie

By seven-fifteen, I'm hovering by the corner of the nurses' station as the ICU staff finish their night shift; Matt is busy taking the final observations, and Jaz is checking drugs. From where I stand the cubicle where Samuel Cox lies is visible, the waveforms on his monitor rising and falling in vivid primary colours. In twelve hours, I've gone from not knowing who he is to having talked to his wife. Last night, Melanie Cox listened to me for a few moments as I introduced myself in a hesitant staccato. Then there was silence. The moment stretched until I heard her voice again, a whisper like a rustle of dead leaves.

When shall we meet? It was as simple as that.

A voice startles me, loud next to my ear. 'What are you doing, Edie? You're not supposed to be here.'

Shit.

My heart pounds, but it's just Jaz. Morris is not due in until eight, but after his ultimatum I'm so nervous about being near the department my pulse is now clattering wildly.

'Jaz, for God's sake.' I suck a breath in. 'I'm just looking. Thinking.'

She follows my gaze to Cox's cubicle. Her lips tighten, her eyes glittering. 'That fucking bastard.'

'Who told you about it?'

'Edie, I didn't mean to pry—'

I shake my head wryly. 'Jaz, everyone knows you can't keep a secret to save your life. You may as well tell me.'

'I tried your mobile an hour ago to ask how you were doing and it went to voicemail, so I phoned Harry. You'd just left.'

'You spoke to Harry?'

'Yeah.' Then, seeing my frustration, 'Don't blame him. He's really concerned about you, honey.' She wraps her arm around my shoulder. 'And so am I.'

'Right. It seems like everyone wants to protect me.'

'No need to be like that. We're there for you, that's all.'

'I know. And thanks, but I'll be okay.'

'I know one thing, Edie: you shouldn't have come into work today. You shouldn't be anywhere near that...' She wrestles with the right word and loses. 'That shitbag over there.'

'He's still a patient, Jaz.'

She snorts. 'Don't give me that medical ethics crap. If I had the guts I'd push a load of fentanyl into the dirty bastard and that'd be the end of it.'

'Wow. I never saw you as a vigilante.'

She sits next to me, still fuming. 'Don't tell me you wouldn't love to do it too.'

'I would, but murder is against the Hippocratic oath,' I tell her. Jaz doesn't smile. As I watch the lines tracing the rhythms of his body, hypnotic in their regularity, I recognise how flat and humourless my voice is. No wonder my attempts at lightening the situation sound misplaced.

'Murder?' Matt has stopped behind us. 'Is it for money or love? Please let it be love, Jaz.' He bats his eyelids theatrically at her.

'Neither,' she snaps. 'Revenge maybe.'

Behind Jaz's back, Matt pulls a scolded face. 'Okay, I get it. So how about you tell me who you want revenge on over a beer after work? I happen to know some reliable hitmen.'

Jaz rolls her eyes. 'Matt, shut up for once. This is a private conversation.'

Matt is one of those people incapable of reading the mood. He squats down between us and whispers slyly. 'So, Doctor Carter, have we found out who this mystery man is yet?'

Jaz glances at me. *I haven't told him.* 'No, not yet, Matt.'

'Oh. Bloody weird though, right?' He waits for someone to speak, eyes wide, but it takes a full half-minute of stony silence for him to get the hint. 'Okay. Well, I'd better go check the resus trolley then, ladies. Last chance, Jaz. I'll even throw in a pizza with that beer.'

'Are you still here?' Jaz tuts, watching him grin and amble away. The profile of her cheek dents with a dimple; she's smiling. 'God, he's more of an old gossip than I am.'

'You like him, don't you?'

'No, he's an idiot.' When Matt is out of sight she swivels on her chair, her smile fading. 'And don't worry, I won't say anything.'

'Jaz, what would you do if you were me?'

'I don't think you want my advice; I think you've made your mind up already.'

'Maybe.'

'I'll support you whatever you do. Either way it's going to cause you pain, Edie, but if that scumbag in there wakes up…' She trails off, frowning. 'Listen, just find out exactly what happened, hon. We can talk it through then, just us. After that, it can't hurt you any more.'

So there's the simple solution, according to Jaz. It was the answer I'd expected from her. She likes things in front of her, out in the light. That's why her relationships until now have always fizzled out, or so she once told me over the third shared bottle of wine; she's too honest. *When they're being a prick,* she'd slurred, *I fucking well tell them.*

'How's his condition?' I ask.

'The same. I reckon if we stopped the anaesthetic, we could take his tube out. It's like Morris wants to stamp his authority.'

'Sometimes I wonder who that guy slept with to get consultant.'

'Euuurgh. That's gross.' Her burst of laughter dies instantly, as she focuses over my shoulder. Someone has walked into the department. Her eyes widen, her grin wilting. As she smooths her scrubs, I know who it is without having to turn. He has arrived early. I should have known.

Mr Punctual, the ultimate control freak. Morris.

When I face him, his eyes bore into mine. His voice is as measured as always. 'Doctor Carter. Five minutes of your time, if you please.'

*

Once again, the drugs cupboard is our makeshift meeting place. At two metres wide and three metres long, it's more of a room than a cupboard, lined with metal units and laminate-covered workbenches that smell faintly of ether. I stand near the row of blood gas analysers and the humming bank of drug and blood fridges, which dominate the far corner. Morris closes the door and stands with his back to it, staring at me in a way that's meant to be intimidating.

I hold his gaze. He doesn't waste any time with niceties.

'What are you doing here?'

'I just needed to pick up some dexamethasone for theatres.' It's such a basic lie he could destroy it in less than five minutes if he wanted to.

'You don't find dexamethasone at the nurses' station. It's been less than twenty-four hours since I asked you not to come into the department.'

Most of my life has felt like an exercise in honing my survival instinct. I can't recall a time when it felt like anything other than me against the world. With my back pressed against the blood fridge, I am now literally cornered. The style of this interrogation has also flicked a switch in me; at the condescending tone of his voice, his arrogance, a cold resentment takes over. I won't be talked to like a child. 'Well, I have questions too, Doctor Morris. Why are you so protective of this patient? Why aren't you extubating? There is no reason to keep him asleep any more.'

'Protective?' He reads my expression and snorts. 'Oh, I see. You've been talking to Jaz. The two of you are inseparable.' Frustrated, he pushes his theatre cap further back on his head. 'She's always been indiscreet. Her head is in the bloody clouds half the time.'

'She's a brilliant nurse. This department would be stuck without her.'

He takes his glasses off and rubs his eyes. 'Just stay away, Edie. I won't ask again.'

I step forward, trying to put myself on the front foot mentally as well as physically.

'You still haven't told me why you haven't extubated.'

'Not that I have to explain myself to you, but he is clearly unstable, possibly psychotic. Therefore, we consider it prudent to delay extubating him.'

'For whose benefit? Mine or yours?'

Morris's eyes flare, his reply hissing through clenched teeth. 'Well, do you want him awake?' He holds my gaze. 'Do you want the man who was disturbed enough to cut your name into his body sitting up and talking? Are you ready for that, Doctor Carter?' He waits. My silence confirms he's touched a nerve.

'You don't have to protect me,' I tell him, my voice steady. 'I already know who he is. I know what he did to me.'

Morris doesn't miss a beat. 'Then all the more reason to keep him asleep.'

'That's unethical.'

'Unethical? It's a valid medical decision, justifiable given his co-morbidities. But don't be hypocritical. Given what he did, I'm sure you don't want him awake either, do you?'

'So now you can read my mind?' Regardless of how accurate his assessment is, I still resent his deciding on my behalf. 'You knew who he was all along, didn't you? How did you find out? My full name wasn't in the newspaper reports.'

'Just listen to me. Keep your appointment with Doctor Wilson this Thursday. Stay away from that man.' He pauses, adjusts his glasses. 'Your primary FRCA exams are in a few months, don't jeopardise them.'

'That sounds like a threat.'

'Call it what you like.' The quick, insincere smile skips across his face again. 'Let me be absolutely clear. If I'm advised that your mental health has suffered because of this patient, and I will be guided by Amy Wilson on this, I will not enter you for your final exams this summer. Neither will I risk the smooth running of this department or bring this hospital any adverse publicity. Understood?'

Everything I want to tell him is bottled up in my throat, like water pressure building behind a creaking, cracking dam. How being controlled makes me want to scream, how his arrogance cuts into me like glass. Instead, I manage another silent nod, barely noticeable.

He glances at his watch. 'And now I suggest you get to theatres; the morning list meeting will be starting soon.'

Just like all the middle-aged, entitled male doctors, he functions best when he's in control. Yes, he accepted me for anaesthetic core training, gave me a chance when some other departments wouldn't. He took me on when all the other Trusts could see were my problems. Rejections passed off with excuses; a poor interview, a very high-quality field, you name it. But now I'm paying for that, and then some. As I pass him, he puts his hand out to stop me. He reaches into one of the cupboards and passes me a handful of blue-and-white boxes with a knowing smile. 'Don't forget these for your list, Edie.'

Dexamethasone, the condescending bastard.

I brush past him, letting him hold onto the belief that I'm back in my box, that he is going to control the way I access my own past. Because he controls my career, he is confident he has me where he wants me. That I'll just go along with his plans.

But I have plans too. And next time, I'll just be more careful.

11

Harry

Josh Bellmore, the man sitting opposite me, is twenty-five. His beard is well-groomed, his mid-brown hair swept into a side parting, and he is outwardly calm and rational. He has been with us for five days, since being talked down from the fourth-floor ledge of the NCP car park in Newhall Street after months of hearing voices telling him the world would be a better place without him in it. As I've been trying to explain to Josh what this episode of psychosis means, Edie's mother has been filling my thoughts. Jenny Carter would have had a similar conversation with her psychiatrist at some point, as she learned that her clinical depression was here to stay. Learned that it can be treated, but not cured. I've met her three times, twice when she was stable enough to be at home, and once when she was a voluntary inpatient at Claydon Manor in North Warwickshire, a private service provider in partnership with the NHS. Each time, all I could see was a patient in extreme denial. Just as Josh is now.

'When am I going home?' he asks.

'Not for a while, Josh.' I keep my reply neutral, as if it's neither a good nor a bad thing. 'How is your mother dealing with it?'

'She doesn't think there's anything wrong with me.'

I nod, smiling my sympathetic psychiatrist smile. Another family member who can't come to terms with what's happening. Another parent unable to deal with the way her child is, and who can blame her? It's Edie and her mother with the roles reversed. When Jenny stops coping, she admits herself to Claydon Manor, and they step in. Willingly, of course, because she's fully insured. Claydon is like a regional version of The Priory, except in Claydon's case the money trickles through to an American investment fund called Valhalla Private Equity. Private capital servicing NHS contracts: it's the sort of setup my father gets all giddy and excited about. As my eyes drift around my NHS office with its chipped, lime-green gloss paint and charity shop furniture, I wonder if he has a point after all.

I show Josh to the door. The haloperidol we put him on is slowly working, and he lets himself be led with a bemused frown. His eyes narrow suspiciously as he surveys the secure unit. 'I'm not happy with this, Doctor Creighton.'

'Hopefully it's not for long, Josh. I'll call your mum again, tell her what's happening.' He wanders along the corridor toward the day room and I flop back down at the desk. That's going to be a tough phone call.

But I have another call to make before Mrs Bellmore, and I've been putting it off ever since I finally decided this morning. Yes, I promised I'd stand by Edie, support her in any way I could. But her idea of helping herself is not the same as mine, and she will need her mother on her side. As I stared into the darkness last night, I realised I had to help Edie the only way I knew how. Is it arrogant to say that she's wrong and I'm right? Maybe, but I can't let her stumble into this alone, led by people who don't understand her the way I do.

Jenny's landline number is on my screen, ready to dial. I press call and put my phone on speaker, tapping my pen nervously, my pulse skittering. I picture the phone ringing in a quiet room, in an empty house. The voice that answers is soft, wary.

'Hello?'

'Jenny? It's Harry. Do you remember me?'

'Edie's Harry?'

There is an edge of anxiety in the higher registers, a brittleness. It's easy now to understand how Jenny's life has been defined by trauma, her uncertain tone honed by years of unimaginable guilt. Hidden in her voice is a remorse so deep that whenever it breaks to the surface, like molten rock hitting the cold air, it must feel as raw as the first time.

'Yeah. How are you?'

'Why are you ringing?'

Seconds pass. The question echoes my sudden sense of doubt, amplifies the uncertainty.

'Jenny, something has happened. I need to talk to you about it.'

'Why? I don't want visitors.'

'Okay, but it's important. It's about what happened to Edie.'

Deep silence again. Has she put the phone down? No, she is still on the line, hardly breathing.

'How do you know what happened?'

'Look, I'd rather tell you in person.'

'How do you know?'

She has become even more defensive, wary. A lioness who has spotted a hunter prowling near her cubs. The shadow of mistrust falls across the sixty miles that separate us.

'Well, the thing is—'

'Harry. Tell me what's happened.'

Now it's my voice that is tentative.

'It's about the man who took her, Samuel Cox. He's in her hospital unconscious, very sick. Edie knows what happened to her, Jenny.'

Silence again. Then a bitter, guarded laugh, as dry as dust.

'Does she? Well, we do our best to protect our children, don't we? Isn't that what parents are supposed to do?'

'Yes, but—'

The voice on the line is a whisper, dripping with self-loathing.

'When you've failed in the one thing you're supposed to do as a mother, where do you go? What do you do?'

'We need your help, Jenny. We need to talk. *Edie* needs to talk.'

'Why are you letting her torture herself? She needs to leave the past alone. We all do.'

'Jenny, I don't think that's possible any more. She needs to understand—'

Then a blast comes from nowhere, an eruption of pent-up anger. Twenty years of guilt bursting from the speaker.

'NO!' Her voice becomes a low, choked growl. 'She needs to let him die.'

'Call ended' flashes on my screen and then the line is dead. What the fuck have I just done?

My office is so silent, even the creaking of my chair is deafening. But it doesn't drown out the gnawing realisation that I have just been guilty of precisely the kind of intrusion that I hate in others. My good intentions mean nothing; instead of putting myself in someone else's position, I've just blundered in. Always the rationalist, I worked on my reasons for doing this until they became the shape I wanted. But in that moment, as Jenny's pain became almost feral, I realised this phone call wasn't about helping, it was about control. About managing the situation.

And I should know because of all the times as a child I was checked up on, spoken about, discussed behind my back. The unwilling subject of all those plans they made. All the times where what was 'right for Harry' had nothing to do with me. When I felt as if I was nothing but a piece in someone else's game. That's what makes the phone call even more of a betrayal. As the logic of why I felt the need to interfere tumbles though my mind, as these questions of motivation stay unanswered, I can feel my muscles tensing in my arms and shoulders, my frustration building. I can dimly hear my own voice repeating a word.

Shit.

Then feel a loud crack, something splintering. I look down and the pen I was holding is in pieces in my fist. I throw the shards at the wall and rub my brow.

I have to keep this call a secret from Edie at all costs. If she found out, it could end us.

And who would blame her? It's the kind of stunt my father has pulled on me all my life, and now I'm doing the same.

Like father, like son, the saying goes.

And that's the most sickening thought of all.

12

Edie

Melanie Cox is pale and drawn, perhaps fifty but looking ten years older, with the pinched, lined mouth of a heavy smoker. She ushers me into a tidy but soulless living room with faded carpet and washed-out beige walls, her hazel eyes scanning me with the guarded look of someone used to hostility. It's impossible to imagine what she must have endured since the trial; the gossip, the stares from her neighbours, the whispers in the street. She motions me to the sofa. It's firm and uncomfortable, barely used.

'Thanks for seeing me, Mrs Cox.'

'I'd prefer it if you'd just call me Melanie.' There are years of shame in her quiet voice. 'I've reverted to my maiden name. It's... you know.'

'Yes, of course. I'm sorry.'

'I'll get you some tea.'

'No, really. You don't have to.'

'It's no trouble.'

As she clatters about in the kitchen, I realise why the room feels so unwelcoming. No photos line the mantelpiece; no pictures hang on the walls. There is nothing personal at all. I briefly wonder why she didn't move away after Cox's conviction. Why stay in this same close-knit Cambridgeshire village, enduring the scandal and rumours? Yet here she is, years later, with a life that has been put on hold. She places a tray on the coffee table, then sits opposite and lights a cigarette.

'Can I be honest, Melanie? I didn't expect you to see me.'

She takes a deep drag before answering. 'I won't pretend your call

67

didn't come as a shock. But I agreed to see you for my own benefit too,' she whispers through a plume of blue smoke, her gaze fixed on the net curtains at the window. 'I'm partly to blame for what he did to you.'

'No. It's not your fault.'

'Yes, it is.' She swivels towards me, cigarette trembling between her close-trimmed nails. 'I should have seen what a sick bastard he was.'

'You mustn't blame yourself. Please, I—'

I'm cut short by another burst of resentment, bitter as a winter squall. 'How can you even stand to be near him? How can you bear to keep him alive?'

'I have to. He's a patient.'

She snorts. 'He's a monster. You, of all people, should know that.'

It's as though she's angry at me for being part of the medical team responsible for saving her ex-husband's life. Part of me can understand that; why wouldn't she be? He's ruined hers after all.

'Melanie, that's the problem. I *don't* know.'

She pulls her cardigan tighter, closing herself off. 'Why are you trying to understand something so… incomprehensible?'

I hesitate, choosing my words. Her trust feels as brittle as glass. 'Look, Samuel chose my hospital for a reason. He had a… message for me.'

'What do you mean?'

'He wants forgiveness.'

'And you're going to give it to him?'

'Melanie, I know how this must sound, but I can't remember what he did to me.'

Her eyes widen, her thin, pencilled brows lift. Doubt, an expression I've become painfully familiar with. I'm reminded of the way Wilson tilts her head as she asks those pointed questions, the way Morris looks at me when we discuss my past.

'How can you not remember someone kidnapping you? Abusing…' She trails off. The smouldering cigarette end burns her fingers, and she crushes it out in the overflowing ashtray.

'It's okay, you can say it.' An unwelcome sensation is rising in me. Frustration? Shame? Moving beneath the surface like a shadow in a dark, unlit sea, some immense creature whose shape I can't quite make out. 'Melanie, I have a condition. It's called dissociative amnesia. I've blocked out the trauma of what happened to me. It may as well have happened to someone else, for all I can remember.'

'Well, isn't it better to forget?'

'No.' My reply is too loud, too quick. I exhale slowly. 'No. It's important for me to know what everyone else seems to know already. Piece it together from what other people remember. I've hidden from it for too long. Do you see?'

'Yes, I suppose so. I'm sorry for what happened to you, Doctor Carter.'

'Thanks, but I don't want pity.'

She gets up to turn the light on as the sun dips behind the houses opposite. In the electric glare, I can see how translucent her skin is, the grey tinge to her lips. I notice the quick, tiny puffs she makes at the end of each breath as she walks, and recognise the early signs of emphysema. She lights another cigarette as she sits down, and I feel a surge of empathy. We've both had to find ways of coping, and who can say whether my version of denial has been any better than hers?

'Do you realise he stalked you for months before he took you?' She is distant again, her voice quiet. 'That he *chose* you?'

'The newspaper reports mentioned it.'

'He had a tough childhood himself, you know. They never mentioned that in the papers, of course. I think he believed suffering was normal. A child isn't born damaged though, is it?'

'No, it isn't.' There's something so lost in her expression, a frown so sad and puzzled, that my voice has thickened with emotion. She's right, children don't just lose themselves. They're always abandoned, let down. Mostly by those they love. And she has searched in vain for a reason to forgive her husband, willed herself to find an explanation, but has ended up hating him more than ever.

'But how many times can you make excuses for someone?' she

continues, oblivious as I recompose myself. 'Lots of kids have tough lives, but they don't abduct people, do they?'

'Melanie, did he say anything to you? Before the abduction?'

She holds my gaze. 'He didn't love me, you know. I think I always understood that, even back then. He had affairs.'

'The reports said you had a child. How did she cope?' As the sentence leaves my lips a barrier drops between us and her eyes become guarded. This is still too raw, so why did I have to push it? I thought I was good at reading people. I backpedal frantically. 'Sorry, I had no right to ask about that. It was your husband I came here to find out about, not your—'

'It doesn't matter. Our daughter is dead, Doctor Carter.'

'Oh. I'm sorry. What was her name?'

'Why does her name matter?' she snaps.

'Sorry.' My stomach lurches. What a clumsy idiot. The conversation has turned and now I'm out of control of the situation, treading water. 'I don't mean to be so insensitive. And please, call me Edie. Doctor Carter sounds so formal.'

'If you don't mind, I'd rather it stayed that way.'

The veil of doubt remains, a thin but impenetrable wall. I try one more time. 'Melanie, please, if you can tell me anything that might help me piece together why he did this…'

For a moment, the room is so silent I can hear the tip of her cigarette crackle as she smokes. Then she laughs, briefly and humourlessly. 'You know, when you rang, I felt I owed you. Isn't that weird?'

'You don't owe me anything.'

'Yes I do. He wrecked my life, and I hate him for it. Guilt ripples out, you see, never ending. It touches everyone.'

I think of my mother and me; how close we once were, and how fractured our lives have become. 'Yes, it does.'

'What I'm about to do will help me as well as you. But I want it understood that I won't ever see you again after this. Do you agree?' She studies my face for a reply and registers my subtle nod. 'Fine. Then maybe it's time to let him tell you what happened in his own words? If you can bear to?'

'He can't talk. He's intubated.'

'I don't mean by speaking.' She eases herself from her chair. 'On the phone I said I had something for you. Follow me.'

As we climb the stairs, her small gasps become quicker with the exertion. The spare bedroom she leads me into looks as though it's never been slept in. She pulls open the door of a small cupboard stacked with boxes.

So she does have memories, she does have photos. Hundreds of them. But the fragments of her past aren't on display. They're hidden here, covered in dust in the dark recesses of an unused room. In front of us is her whole life, thrown into packing boxes, as if she'd been waiting to move away for the last twenty years.

From a small box near the back, she pulls a plain black journal. Her fingers brush the cover with something that might have once been affection. 'I found this long after his conviction. Don't ask me why I kept it.'

'What is it?'

'His diary. You wanted to know what sort of man he was. So take it.'

I don't know how long I hold the journal, staring at it, before I open the cover. It feels like a long time in the silence of the vacant bedroom. Inside, Cox's writing is neat and careful. It doesn't look like the ramblings of a deranged mind, but then sociopaths are rarely wild-eyed maniacs. I flick through the yellowing pages; the writing stops on 27 June 2004, the day before my abduction.

'Have you read it?' I ask.

'Some. Not much.' She wipes her eyes angrily as she closes the box and shuts the cupboard door. 'I don't want to hate him any more than I already do. But it might help you remember.'

'Perhaps reading it could give you some closure?'

'Closure? There isn't any. Not for me.' She shrugs and forces a thin smile, in that moment looking older than ever. 'And there won't be for you, either.'

13

Edie

Melanie is getting suspicious, I'm out of the house all hours now. E is more than an obsession. I am neglecting my own family for the sake of watching her. It looked like she had fresh bruises today on her arm. How does nobody else notice this?

At first, I just watched her from afar; I would watch her across the school playground, where she would stand alone, never joining in with the others when they played, and it broke my heart. I wanted to hold her, tell her I could make it better. As an excuse to see E, I made a habit of doing the school run with my daughter — it's okay for a man to hang around the school gates when he has a child in tow. As long as the men have a reason to be there, we mostly get ignored by the women who cluster together. But I still got a reputation as a loner in my dishevelled jogging bottoms and hoodie, and the mothers remained fiercely protective, giving me suspicious glances. But just for those five minutes, I could watch her. Standing apart from the rest, I would wave into the playground, as if catching my daughter's eye, but she was off playing with her friends and didn't notice me. Even my own daughter has grown cold to me lately, just like Melanie. Mel is turning her against me. I know it, but I can't stop doing this. I can't let it go.

E would always be at the far edge of the playground tarmac where no other kids went, kicking her shoe along the painted lines, her pink schoolbag slung over her shoulder. When kids ran past, screaming and laughing, I could see her flinch. She hated loud noises, she was jumpy. She didn't look at the other children directly; instead she would tilt her head and watch them sidelong as they played. What was going through her mind? Did she secretly want to join in? I never let her see me, but I'd watch her until the school bell rang, and she followed the other children inside. Always the last to go in. And when her small figure had disappeared into the corridor, I would leave.

But now, there are no more school gates for me. Melanie does the school run these days. I don't know if people complained about the way I was staring at E; thought I was strange, perhaps? Who could blame them? Maybe it's just another way for Melanie to turn the knife. But it's proven one thing: I'm resourceful. I've found other ways of tracking her to and from school without being noticed.

I've found other ways of watching her.

May 12th 2004

There are garages near her house, and I park there whenever I can, looking at the closed curtains. I watch the lights going on and off, people moving from room to room, wondering what is happening inside. Sometimes a low light will go on in her room, way past the bedtime of an eight-year-old girl. There will be a shadow at the curtains.

Why am I so certain she is unhappy? Because I know the signs.

I'm watching you, E. Looking out for you.

God, if they only knew the truth.

Why shouldn't I watch her? I have every right to follow a child if I think she's in trouble, especially her. I can't keep watching it happen indefinitely, though. I can't see her going through this for much longer. The main problem is keeping what I'm doing discreet. I know they're getting worried about me at work; I've had too many days off sick. I'll probably lose my job if this carries on. But I know how it feels for a child to be scared. Only I know how she feels.

I've seen the bruises, I've seen her fear. The quiet watchfulness. She doesn't trust adults, and why would she? The way other people have missed this is unforgivable. The way they all stay silent is contemptible. All the people who are supposed to be on her side have let her down. Not *me, though. But what's been happening to her that I don't know about? I've done my best; I've made notes, I've marked times and dates, thinking that soon I'm going to report it. But I know I never will. No one is going to believe me. And it would ruin everything. It would ruin everyone. It would all come out then, and there would be no more secrets. There would be no winners. I have no choice; this is for me to deal with alone.*

So now I watch her. In the morning, at night, whenever I can. I park in quiet places, I watch the windows. Does her light still come on at unusual hours? Is he at home with her? I can't bear to think about it. I can't just add her name to all the ones who slip through the net because no one did anything. All those like me. I can't let her feel the way I did.

'Hey, gorgeous.'

A low voice hisses in my ear, making me jump. Jesus, Harry. My heart hammering, I feel his arms snake around my waist from behind, and I'm back at the table in our warm, low-lit kitchen. Next to me, my coffee has gone cold. He kisses me on the back of my neck, but I pull away, twisting towards him.

'You nearly gave me a heart attack.'

He picks up the diary and flicks through it. 'Lost in the ramblings of a madman, were you?'

I'd texted him about the diary when I arrived home. A large part of me had wanted to throw it in the grate, light it and watch it burn. I'd spent an hour wrestling with the same blend of revulsion and curiosity as Melanie Cox must have known for years. Unlike her, though, my curiosity had won.

'A madman?' I shake my head. 'How professional of you. It's obvious from this he's damaged. From childhood, probably.'

'Edie, he abducted someone. *You*, in fact. He confessed to abusing you. Even if you can't remember it, why are you defending him?'

'I'm not. I'm just saying, he could have been abused himself as a kid. Who knows? Give me the child at seven, right?'

'Yeah. And I'll give you an adult with an excuse.'

As Harry scans the pages, my irritation grows. This is not his; he doesn't have the same right as me to read Cox's words. As I read the diary, I could almost touch the loneliness. Harry is sucking his lip distractedly as he reads.

'What do you know about suffering anyway?' I ask. He doesn't reply so I plough on, trying to draw him out of his detached indifference to Cox's pain. 'Be honest, you haven't had to overcome a single obstacle in your life.'

Before he drops his gaze to the journal again, a flash of resentment flits across his face.

'I see. You're psychoanalysing me now?'

'What do you think?'

'I think I know plenty about suffering.' He drops onto a stool at the kitchen island and drags a hand through his hair. When he eventually looks up, the frown is gone, and he is looking at me through the same open, guileless eyes that I fell in love with. He holds the journal up like a courtroom exhibit. 'And this should have gone to the police, by the way.'

'She didn't find it until years after his conviction.'

'Yeah, but it was new evidence. I'm no detective, but even I know that.'

'Who knows what she was thinking? You should have seen her.'

'All right.' He sighs loudly. 'But I don't understand why you're putting yourself through this.'

'What else do you suggest?'

'Burn the fucking thing. Take some sick leave until this guy either dies—' he crosses his fingers in a *let's hope* gesture '—or survives and gets rearrested. Quit your sessions with Wilson. I told you, she's a quack. Trust me, I know. I have to work with her, remember? She's indiscreet, unprofessional. She *shares* too much.'

'Does she realise you badmouth her every chance you get?'

Harry shrugs ruefully. 'Come on, it's true. She's useless. You've said so yourself.'

'Okay. But if it wasn't for Morris insisting on those sessions, you and I might never have met.'

'True.' He stares at the diary in his hand. 'Listen, final offer. Let me get rid of this for you, Edie. It's not helpful.'

'I thought you wanted to support me?'

'I do.'

'Then let me do things my way.' I grab for the book and it falls on the table, sending my coffee slopping across the surface. 'Oh, shit.'

Harry ignores the brown puddle. 'Edes? Look.'

I follow his gaze to the diary. He is holding the rear cover open, with one finger just above a slit in the pasted-down endpaper. A small triangle of colour is showing, a sharp corner, with the grainy texture and unmistakable sheen of a photograph. He works the slit open, revealing more of the picture, little by little.

Yellow, sun-washed sand. A purple jelly shoe, a child's leg.

I take the diary from him, working the picture out of the pocket it had been hidden in. Two girls on a beach are posing theatrically, smiling. They are seven or eight, with matching star-shaped sunglasses, swimsuits and hair glistening wet as if they'd just run from the sea, their arms draped across each other's shoulders. They could almost be sisters. It takes me a while to understand what I'm seeing. I'm barely aware of Harry's hand gently squeezing my shoulder. As I gaze at the glossy, six-by-four photo, I realise that I'm staring at myself. My own gap-toothed smile, my green swimsuit. I can feel its wetness on me. I remember everything about it, from the shellfish pattern to the way the shoulder straps rubbed when they got sand under them.

The photo draws me in. The gentle pressure of Harry's hand becomes the weight of the other girl's arm across my back as we hug. I can sense her touch, but the rest of her is vague. As the photograph fills my vision, as I move closer, even the sounds from this captured moment in time drift towards me from some shadowed, hidden corner of my mind. Gulls are calling as they wheel and soar above the bay behind us. The noises of a beach in summer rise up from somewhere inside me; laughter, the sound of the ocean, our squeals as we run away from the waves. I can feel them crashing over us as the sea catches up, pushing us over. There is the smell of seaweed on the sand, and the tang of saltwater drying on our skin. The sun is warm on my back, and on her back too. Her closeness feels good somehow; I've missed it. The door opens briefly in my mind, and she and I are in the blue sea, drifting up and down as if we're riding the tide.

I chase the memory, but it slips out of reach. My fingers trace the lines of my face, the other girl's face. We are not scared; we are content. We are just children.

'Edes? Are you okay?'

My voice sounds as though it's coming from somewhere else. 'Why has he got this photo, Harry? How did he get it?'

Harry's voice is quiet, shocked. 'Edie. Look on the back.'

He turns the photograph over. On the white surface, where the faded brand name of the film is stamped, something is written in Biro. Three words and a date.

Edie and Sophie, July 2003.

The writing doesn't match Cox's, but it is still familiar. The letters slope forward, curly and expressive. The tails are looped, the distinctive double-storey of the letter *a*. The i of Edie is dotted with a small heart. Yes, it's unmistakably hers.

I'd know my mother's handwriting anywhere.

14

Harry

The Saturday morning traffic on the M6 has added half an hour onto our journey as we leave Birmingham, heading towards Northampton. It's been good thinking space, but a way of admitting to Edie what I've done still hasn't presented itself. I'm going to be forced to wing it, but I'm finding her mood impossible to judge because we haven't spoken since leaving Harborne. She's in her own world, as remote from me as if we're travelling in different cars. An hour and a half ago, she'd slid the photo into the inside pocket of her jacket and shoved the diary in her bag. It was hard to tell whether her expression was decisiveness or fear as she'd grabbed the car keys. I'd stalled for time, trying to give us space to talk.

'So you're just going to turn up at your mum's house, and push this photo under her nose?'

'It's her writing, Harry. I've got no other option, have I? Unless you have a better idea?' *No*, I thought, *I'd had a far worse idea in phoning your mother myself.* She'd stared at the keys, twisting the keyring through her fingers like a worry bead. 'To be honest, I'd rather you didn't come.'

'Edie, please. I'm coming. If you insist on seeing her, then I need to be there to support you.' While this was true, I could only bear to be so hypocritical about the phone call because I was trying to save my own skin, although it was obvious that, in the next few hours, the truth was going to come out one way or another. I'd eventually persuaded Edie to let me drive there, using the fact that the visit might upset her as an excuse, so at least I could be there to explain when the shit finally hit the fan. White lies are much easier to rationalise, aren't they?

The village of Stoke Bruerne is on the Grand Union Canal, and people have descended on it from what feels like the whole county to take advantage of the warm spring weather. The canal bridge is decked out in red, white and blue bunting, and music plays from one of the moored boats where four white-haired men have set up an impromptu 1940s band. Snatches of 'In the Mood' reach the car as we cross the bridge, the people below us milling around the pub and canal-side, where stalls are selling *bric-à-brac* and cakes. Edie doesn't notice any of it; we are only a few streets from her mother's cottage, and she has the fixed, tense expression of a bomb disposal expert who has forgotten which wire to clip.

'I hate these twee little places,' she manages, her voice low. 'Give me the city any day.'

'Edes, do you want me to go in and see her first?' I ask. To prepare the ground, of course, how gallant of me.

'No. Visiting my mother these days is like ripping a plaster off. It's better to just get on with it.'

Jenny Carter's cottage is in a small terrace of Victorian two-up, two-downs, probably old canal workers' houses. We park the car at the end of the narrow street and walk the twenty yards to her door. Edie knocks, but, whatever emotions are simmering away, she now has them under control. She has her doctor's face on: detached, professional, aloof.

Then the door swings open, and she is face to face with her mother for the first time in a year. I haven't seen Jenny for even longer. She is smaller than I remember, and her hair is greyer and thinner, maybe a side effect of her medication. As she looks at us both, recognition gradually oozing across her face, I smile at her with a mute appeal to keep quiet about our phone call. Without a word, she leaves the door open, and we follow her into a small, overheated front room, with a log burner and big worn armchairs, and cluttered with ornaments. Through a low arch at the far end, an oak table sits near a pair of French doors leading to the garden. Edie leans down to Jenny and they kiss awkwardly. Jenny busies herself, clearing some space on the table.

'It's been a long time since I last saw you, Edie,' she says to the floor, eyes down.

Edie puts a hand on her shoulder. 'I know, I'm sorry. How have you been?'

'I'm coping. I like it here.'

Jenny passes me on her way to the kitchen. She glances at me, her mouth pinched. She doesn't trust me; perhaps it's my psychiatrist's bearing. But at that glance I relax, as my instinct tells me she won't mention the call. It's as if she feels it was none of my business in the first place. Edie follows her to the kitchen door and I wait in the front room, listening.

'Mum, I need to speak to you.'

'What about?'

'Samuel Cox.' She pauses. 'Mum, he's come back.'

'Has he?' Jenny pushes past her and sits at the table. Something flickers in her eyes, too brief to place, then her lines deepen in a frown and the barrier is up again. A shaft of sunlight breaking through the tall French doors washes her face and she looks ten years older. 'It was only a matter of time, wasn't it?'

'Why are you so calm? Don't you know what this means?'

Jenny smiles wearily, showing uneven teeth. 'Of course. As I said, only a matter of time.'

I am grateful for my invisibility now, for the fact neither of them seem to know I'm here. They're skirting around each other like boxers, neither of them allowing the other one near. Jenny's eyes remain fixed on the table as Edie sits opposite her. She slides the journal from her bag, then fishes in her pocket and drops the photograph face-up in front of her mother.

'Mum, who is this?'

Jenny looks up, eyes fixed on her, ignoring the photo. 'Do you want some tea?'

Edie stabs the photo. 'No, thanks. I want you to tell me what you remember about this.'

'Harry, would you like something to drink?'

Edie takes her mother's hand, dragging her attention away from me. 'Mum, who's the girl in the photo?'

'It's you, my darling.'

'No, the other girl.'

'Nobody. A friend?'

I thought Edie was composed, but I was wrong. Her questions are tumbling out; she is hardly waiting for answers. It is like an interrogation. She turns the photo over. 'I found this in Samuel Cox's diary. It's your writing on the back. Why did he have it?'

Jenny shakes her head, wisps of hair catching the sunlight. 'I don't know who wrote that.'

'Why did he have the photo?'

'Who?'

'You know who.'

Finally, Jenny picks up the photograph like a specimen, holding it by the corner. The paper shakes, exaggerating the mild tremor in her hand. I try to calculate what medication she is on. Fluoxetine? Sertraline? She seems calm, unfazed, but not over-sedated.

'It's not my writing.' Jenny drops the photo onto the table again next to the journal. 'Please my love, just let it go.'

'Mum, why has Cox come back? I want to hear it from you. What exactly did he do?'

'Read the newspapers. They don't print lies.' A faint light shines in Jenny's eyes. A glimmer of something powerful enough to poke its way through the warm, medicated blanket she's under. Then, a scowl twists her face. 'How I wish that bastard was dead.'

'Mum, I'm sorry if it feels like I'm interrogating you. But it *is* your writing. So how did Cox get it? Who's the other girl?' Edie leans closer, her hand on her mother's arm, enclosing it. Her voice is insistent, verging on desperate. 'You've protected me for years, but I need to know now. Please, tell me what you remember.'

Jenny won't hold her daughter's gaze; she looks beaten somehow. Her lips move, making soundless words as she stares at the tablecloth.

'Edie, don't do this,' I whisper. Perhaps part of me is trying to make up for the shock I gave this poor woman by calling her. 'You're upsetting her.'

My voice breaks the tension between the two women. As Edie turns towards me, relaxing her grip, Jenny's sudden movement takes us both by surprise. She snatches the photo and begins tearing at it, the pieces dropping on the table like confetti. Edie, reacting just as quickly, grabs the pieces and the diary, before Jenny can tear into that as well.

Edie stares at the fragments, her hands shaking. 'What did you do that for?'

Her mother sits back in her armchair, breathless, then turns away, staring out of the window. 'I don't remember anything,' she hisses, glancing between Edie and me as if proving it to us both. 'Are you satisfied now? I just don't remember.'

'Okay, Mum, just calm down,' Edie says, but Jenny's gaze has already drifted out to the garden again.

'Edie, I'm sorry,' she whispers. Tears begin rolling down her cheek, catching the light as she stares through the window at nothing.

'It's okay.' Edie glances down at the photo fragments. 'Don't cry.'

Even though we're all sitting at the same table, I'm still excluded. These two women are remote from me, and their connection is beyond my understanding. I'm not a real part of this, and I never will be; I'll only ever be on the fringe of their relationship. Whatever has passed between them in the past is not for me to know. Maybe that's why I have the urge to moderate, to be a peacemaker. Or maybe it's just because I'm frightened that at any moment they'll begin tearing each other apart.

'Edie, come on,' I say. 'You're just upsetting each other. SSRI medication often affects memory; maybe she really doesn't remember.'

Jenny turns back from the window and watches us both. Her eyes dart between us, her movements bird-like, fidgety. 'Yes, he's right. I don't remember. So why don't you both leave me alone? This has come as a shock.'

'Let's go, Edes. Sorry to have upset you, Mrs Carter.' She doesn't acknowledge me. I get up and offer her my hand, but it hovers in the air until I drop it lamely to my side. I wait for Edie to follow, but the two women are immobile, holding each other's eyes. The atmosphere is heavy. I can tell they want me to leave them and I'm happy to oblige. I stroke Edie's back. 'I'll be in the car.'

I'm at the front door when I hear it. Her mother's thin, querulous voice, somehow both low and sharp at the same time. Through the crack in the door, I can see a glimpse of the table. They are standing now, close to each other, and Jenny is looking at Edie with penetrating, razorblade clarity. The older woman is several inches shorter and has craned her neck, pulling her jaw tight as she leans towards her daughter. Jenny doesn't know I'm still here; this isn't meant for me. This is between the two of them, and no one else.

'It ruined my life,' she whispers to her daughter, her voice cracking, carrying in the silence. 'And if you don't let this go, it will ruin yours too.'

15

Edie

Routine urology lists might not be glamorous, but they're fast and unrelenting. The day flies and you don't get time to dwell on anything. Twelve procedures a day. The patient comes into the anaesthetic room and I check their details, then it's cannulate, IV propofol, laryngeal mask, into theatres to watch cantankerous surgeon Bob Stoneham do his thing, and then wheel the sleeping patient into recovery. Rinse and repeat. But work hasn't completely pushed the visit to my mother from my mind. Every time I've taken an elderly patient's hand to look for a vein, it's my mother's frail bones and crepe-paper skin I touch again. Every nervous patient's eyes are hers, as she begs me not to rake up the past. She has lost the strength to keep going, and feels like an old woman to me already. Only fifty-four, but done with life.

The journey home had been as silent as the one going, with Harry and I both wrapped in our thoughts. He'd looked shell-shocked in the car after my mother's sudden attack on the photograph, and maybe now he'll understand why I don't like to visit her. I can still see him open-mouthed as she shredded the picture, which I spent half an hour repairing when we got home. At least he wasn't there to hear her whispered threat at the end. It unnerved me at first, but then I rationalised it. She is more vulnerable than me, more easily rattled. All week I've pictured her pacing around the empty house, fretting, scaring herself, pushing it all away as usual, whereas I see this as something we can't ignore any more. I knew I was risking triggering her, but what else could I do? She knew him somehow, and I had to see what she would say. But then yesterday, I got the inevitable call from Claydon Manor.

As she might have said herself, it was only a matter of time.

I'd recognised Sue Willard's voice immediately from one of my mother's previous visits to the unit. Willard is the senior sister and has the perfect bureaucratic tone of voice to fit her role; she is superficially polite – my mother is a paying client, after all – but has the dogmatic manner and condescending pitch that suggests she'll make life difficult unless you do things her way. *Doctor Carter*, she'd trilled, *I rang to let you know your mother is with us again. She has requested an inpatient stay, and, luckily, we could accommodate her.* Perfectly matter-of-fact, apart from the subtle tone of accusation, the slight hint of blame in her clipped, prissy manner. What kind of daughter allows this to happen to her mother? Where is the support? Well, screw you, Willard, you don't have a clue about us. I'd kept my cool and told her I'd let my mother settle before visiting. *Of course, Doctor Carter*, she declared, as if it was obvious such a neglectful daughter wouldn't bother making the trip immediately.

Harry and I have danced around the whole subject, as though there is a tacit agreement to let things lie. We've spent our evenings at home talking about nothing. The weather, the traffic, which Netflix series to watch next. But Cox's presence is still there, a ghost in the room, and nothing is settled. Far from it. Alone in the kitchen, I've often taken the picture out and examined it, mining it for information, interrogating it. The girls, now with clear tape across their faces, beam back at me. We were close, I can sense it. My crooked, goofy smile, and our bodies merging as our arms drape around each other, bring something warm into the darkness when I imagine myself at that age.

At the KG, as soon as I'm in scrubs, I hover outside the ICU until I see Jaz. I beckon her over, realising how much I've missed talking to her in the last couple of days. She gives me a brief, harassed hug.

'Jaz, can we meet later? I want to talk. I've got some things on my mind.'

She nods. 'Sure. I was worried – why haven't you rung me? You're my best friend, Edie. What happened to sharing things?'

'I know, I'm sorry. I've just been keeping my head down, trying not to think too much. It hasn't worked, though. Anyway, I didn't want to drag your mood down too.'

She utters a theatrical groan of frustration. 'The only thing that'll get me down is *not* talking. I want to help. That's what I'm here for.'

I smile my thanks. 'I've been making every excuse possible to get into the department when Morris isn't around. From borrowing equipment to loitering around emergency theatres in case we have to transfer someone. I've been desperate to find out how Cox is doing.'

'You've been hanging around the department? Morris will go ape. Edie, do you want a career here or not?'

'ICU is part of the hospital, Jaz. I can't be expected to avoid it completely. So how is the patient?'

'Still improving, but still intubated. I'll tell you more later. When do you want to meet?

I do some mental calculations. A full list. The session with Wilson. 'How does seven at The Five Bells sound? I'm going to need a drink after spending an hour with the ice queen.'

'I bet.' She kisses me on the cheek. 'All right, see you there. Got to dash, Fiona's called in sick.'

'Again? That woman's never in.' Jaz nods, rolls her eyes and trots back towards the ICU. 'Jaz,' I call. She stops and turns. 'Thanks,' I say, feeling a little awkward. She shrugs and blows me a kiss, then she's gone.

The Five Bells is a dive of a pub opposite the hospital and will be filled with frazzled junior doctors and nurses on a Friday night. Jaz and I can find a table out of the way somewhere. At least she is someone I can talk to honestly. I don't have the same bond with anyone else. Actually, I don't have anyone else to talk to, period. There's Harry, but he's male and therefore doesn't count. Not in that way. The depressing fact is, I have acquaintances in my life but no real female friends except Jaz. What a sad case I am.

As soon as I walk into Amy Wilson's office, I sense trouble. Wilson is at her desk as usual, but flanking her are Morris and a woman I've never met. Morris's eyes and mine lock as I pause at the doorway.

The woman is creeping towards fifty but trying to be thirty, and her whole aura screams management, from her black cashmere business suit to her salon-perfect makeup.

I hesitate. 'Oh sorry, should I…?' The sentence hangs. Should I do what? Wait outside? Come back later? Run screaming?

'Ah, come in, Doctor Carter.' Morris beckons me forward, and I ease my way into the room. The three look like an interview panel, and I fight the urge to be deferential. I sit straight-backed before them and meet their eyes, one by one. Morris waves a languid hand toward the woman. 'This is Dawn Simpson – she's from HR.'

'Okay,' I venture warily.

The woman's smile is thin, closed-mouthed and, in my current mood, it feels predatory. My heart drops into my shoes; this is about my final exams. Morris is going to defer me, or, worse, recommend I leave core training. As always, when I feel threatened, I go on the offensive.

'Do I need my union rep here?'

'No, no, no.' Her voice is neutral, used to meetings like this. 'Doctor Morris has just asked me to sit in, that's all. Moderate, if you will.'

'Dawn has been informed of the situation, Edie,' purrs Morris. My first name always sounds jarring coming from him, and he notices my frown. 'I hope you don't mind.'

'Edie—' Wilson leans forward '—this is a difficult time for everyone. For you, for Richard, for the hospital as a whole. We need to have a consensus on how we will handle this.'

'I thought it was already being handled?' I keep my expression as flat as possible. 'I've agreed to stay in theatres away from Samuel Cox while Doctor Morris treats him.' I want to add the word 'badly' to the end of the sentence, but resist.

Morris sighs. 'Yes, but you haven't been staying away, have you?'

'I've only visited the department when necessary.'

'That's not what we've heard.'

I glance at Dawn Simpson; she's making notes. 'Heard? From whom?'

'That's not important.'

'Matt?' I scan their faces. Nothing. A deep, gnawing twinge of betrayal twists my stomach. No, it can't be Jaz, surely. She wouldn't.

'As I said, it's not important.' Morris leans forward. 'You are not engaging with us, Doctor Carter. Not prepared to meet us halfway.'

'Walking out of our session last week was another example,' Wilson pitches in.

The woman from HR tries to soften her expression. 'Edie, I can only imagine how difficult this must be for you, but Doctor Morris and Doctor Wilson are trying to help you. We know how you must feel.'

The sympathetic curve of her smile is too much for me. 'Excuse me, but what do you know about how I feel? Anyway, I thought you were just here to moderate?'

Wilson glances at her as if to say, *see, I told you she was difficult.* I can feel this meeting slipping away from me. I'm in a kangaroo court where the verdict is already decided.

Morris's next sentence confirms it.

'Edie, we think you need some time away from the hospital.'

'No, I want to work. It keeps me from…' I breathe hard. 'It keeps my mind occupied.'

'I'm sorry,' he continues, still frowning, 'but you need to be away from this man.'

'Why? Samuel Cox doesn't scare me.' The words come out in an angry flood before I can filter them. 'Maybe you believe he should, but he doesn't.'

'Have you found out any more about him since he arrived?' Wilson's tone is now that of someone talking to a difficult child. 'Have you been investigating him?'

'Like you've been investigating me, Amy?' I turn towards the HR woman. 'Perhaps you should ask yourself how *that* feels, Ms Simpson?'

Wilson remains implacable. 'Well, have you?'

'No.' The lie comes easily. 'But I do think you lot are more scared of him than I am.'

'Okay…' Morris stands. 'I can see that nothing we're saying is making a blind bit of difference.'

'Hold on,' I snap, indignant. 'So you can take an interest in my past, but I can't? How does that work?'

'Calm down, Edie,' Wilson murmurs.

'I am calm,' I hiss at her. 'But you need to tell me what you know about me. If I'm going to be compliant, you need to tell me how much *you've* found out.'

Wilson glances at Morris, who nods for her to continue. The look they share is conspiratorial. 'We know all about your abduction, as you know. How we found out is not important. We know you were traumatised. We won't go into details for obvious reasons. We also know your mother is suffering with depression and is an occasional voluntary inpatient at a private facility.'

My stomach knots. I think of Willard's phone call. 'How do you know that?'

'Edie, clinical psychiatry is a small world. You're a doctor, you treat patients, so we have made it our business to know about anything that might affect your mental… stability. You can understand that, surely?'

Morris takes over, like a tag team. 'Cox was abused in prison; we have spoken to the mental health team at Wakefield where he was held. He was constantly attacked by other prisoners, and yet he never asked for special protection.'

'You've really done your homework.'

'It's simply more evidence of how unstable he might be if he wakes.'

He's lying, I can see it in his eyes. He's a control freak, and I've been played like a fish on a line. And if it's not manipulation, then why take such an interest in my past? There's something behind both his and Wilson's professional detachment that tells me I'm being micromanaged to perfection.

'So when *are* you going to wake him?' I keep my voice as measured as his, glancing at Dawn Simpson. 'Whenever suits you?'

'No,' Morris interjects, standing. 'When it's clinically safe. This is my department, Edie. You know I will not allow it to be disrupted.'

89

'Having spoken to Doctor Morris, I agree,' Dawn Simpson states, business-like once more. 'You shouldn't be anywhere near this man when he wakes.'

'There's a surprise,' I hiss through my teeth.

She hears but doesn't miss a beat. 'Doctor Wilson has assured me that scenario would be catastrophic for your mental health.'

'*My* mental health? Do you realise how condescending that is?'

Morris, still standing, exchanges a glance with her, then sits on the edge of the desk, facing me. 'Edie, this is getting us nowhere. You're on compassionate sick leave, one month. Your FRCA exam dates are safe for now. That's the deal, I'm afraid.'

'Fine.' I feel anything but fine as I get up to leave. My heart is pounding, but I'm trying to keep my exterior calm. At medical school, it's known as the swan: paddling away like mad underneath, gliding along serenely on the surface. 'Thanks for showing how little trust you all have in me.'

Having the last word is the one small victory they allow me. I keep my composure all the way through the musty corridors and out into the cool late afternoon air. Then I'm out in the car park again and letting out a primal yell of powerless, frustrated anger.

They don't want me involved? Okay.

Whatever they know about my past, they're keeping secret. My mother has run for the sanctuary of Claydon Manor, scared to talk about it.

So I'll just have to find it out for myself.

16

Edie

The Five Bells pub only survives financially because it's next to the hospital and for decades has been a convenient place for stressed NHS staff to let off steam. It doesn't look like it has been refurbished since the 1970s, and the décor still carries the ghosts of all those long-gone student nurses and doctors who smoked and drank their way through training. This place must have lost count of the break-ups, breakdowns and illicit love affairs it has hosted over the years. The saloon bar is busy and loud as always, and through the crowd I spot Jaz in the corner. I've already texted Harry to say I'm going to be late, so I snake my way to her table. She's bought a bottle of white and two glasses, thank God. I silently pour myself a full glass and finish it in one long swallow before refilling.

'Bastards.' I wipe my mouth and finally meet Jaz's amused stare.

'I knew there was something I liked about you, Doctor Carter.' Jaz pours herself a glass. 'I think it's your quiet, reserved nature.'

'Give me time for another glass or two and I won't be so polite.' I take another drink, letting its calming effect soothe me. 'They've put me on sick leave. I'm not in the right state of mind to cope, apparently.'

The smile disappears from Jaz's face, replaced by a wide-eyed concern. 'Are you serious?'

'They say having Samuel Cox in the department is bad for my mental health.'

'Oh, Edie.' Jaz chews her lip. She'll be looking for positives. 'Okay, but have you considered they might have a point? A few weeks away is better than getting pulled from your training completely, right?'

'No, I don't see it that way. It's just not right at all that I should be made to take leave.'

Jaz sighs and tops my already half-empty glass up again. 'I know, honey. And I understand that work sometimes keeps us both sane. You know how I feel about this job; it saved me and I'd be lost without it. It gave me purpose, direction.'

'Yeah, I know.' She's right. We've talked about this a lot. Jaz getting onto nurse training pulled her out of a trough in her life so deep she couldn't see a way of climbing out. I was the same before this career. I was just coping. Medicine forces you to think of other people and gives you perspective in a way nothing else does, and we'd both be lost without it. She reads my mind.

'We're the same, me and you. This job is part of who we are. So I do understand, Edie, honestly. But maybe it's time to just give yourself some headspace?'

'I don't know, Jaz.'

'Come on, think of yourself. Maybe some time away might be a good idea. You try not to show it, but the last week must have really messed with you.'

'Delicately put.' I briefly resent her making the same assumption as Morris and Wilson. 'I know I shouldn't have hung around the department, but I couldn't help myself.'

'You're right, you shouldn't have. This sicko abused you, Edie.'

A drunk guy heading towards the fruit machine bumps into our table with a low, slurred apology. Jaz shoots him an angry glare. In the last couple of weeks, it has felt like I'm losing the ability to judge people, and my sense of being cut adrift has deepened. In the noise of the pub, a wave of loneliness engulfs me.

'So why aren't I afraid of him then?' I venture, watching her expression. 'Wilson is always going on about how dissociative amnesia leaves residual feelings behind. Fear, hatred. If so, why aren't I scared?'

'I don't know, Edie,' she shrugs. 'But I do know it's okay to hate him. He hasn't exactly earned your forgiveness, has he?'

I glance at the guy on the fruit machine, but he's taking no notice of us, glassy eyes hypnotised by the spinning reels. 'I'm not even sure what to forgive. Everything feels like it's closing in right now, Jaz. Do you want me to be honest?'

'Of course.'

'It feels like everyone wants me out of the way. Like I'm an inconvenience.'

The silence that follows is punctuated by the manic, babbling music of the machine, as the guy pumps money in. Jaz leans closer. 'Edie, that sounds a bit paranoid, if you don't mind me saying.'

She doesn't need to tell me that. I've been wrestling with it for years. It never goes away. Am I as good as the other students? Will my background go against me? Are they talking about me? Low self-esteem takes so much energy to camouflage. 'Maybe,' I reply eventually. 'What are people in the department saying?'

'Nothing, really. People are discreet.'

'Jaz, maybe you're right and I'm overthinking this, but you know how I am. It feels horrible being left outside. I need to know what's going on in the hospital.'

'Do I sense a favour coming on?' Jaz smiles wryly, way ahead of me.

'Well? Would you? Be my eyes and ears in the department.'

'Spy, you mean?'

'It's not exactly spying, is it? I just want you to keep me informed about Cox's condition.' I pause, knowing how she'll react to my next sentence. 'Jaz, I've spoken to his wife.'

'God, Edie, are you mad?'

'No, but there's more to this than meets the eye. I feel like I have a stake in this but am being left out by Morris.'

'I meant to tell you. He pulled me in for one of his chats the other day, had a go at me for letting Matt show you the unknown patient. He seemed to think it was all my fault.'

'He's good at blaming people by proxy. He knows we're friends. To be honest, I think it's one of the reasons he wants me off work for a while. He wants me away from you as well.'

'Well, maybe he's right, hon. Not about us, but about work. This situation isn't healthy for you. You seem…'

Healthy. There's that word again. As she trails off, I empty the bottle into our glasses.

'Go on, you can tell me. You're supposed to be a friend.'

'I am a friend. Well, you're getting fixated. Obsessed. I've never seen this side of you before.'

A flush of indignation touches my cheeks, but only because I know she's right. I sip my wine, collecting my thoughts, still on edge from the meeting. Nobody knows what it's like to bury a secret so deep you can't even face it yourself. You're incomplete. Unfinished, somehow. None of them can see what it means to be hurt so badly your own consciousness won't let you deal with it. Your mind working as an enemy, hiding things from you. And as for others knowing? That's the worst part of all, because I will be judged regardless, despite no one understanding it. How can anyone understand? It hasn't happened to *them*. If I'm paranoid, I have every right to be. The stakes are too high for me to be any other way.

'Okay,' I finally say, and nod, reluctantly. 'I get it. If enough people say it's time to take a step back, who am I to argue?'

Jaz reaches for my hand. 'Look, I'll keep you informed about what's going on at the KG, Edie. I promise. Just take time for yourself, okay?' She looks wistfully at the empty bottle and then checks her watch. 'I wish we had time for another couple. I don't like rushing off like this.'

'It's only eight, so why can't we? I'm getting a cab home.'

She checks her phone, distracted, then drops it in her bag. 'Much as I'd love to, I'm meeting a guy in the Jewellery Quarter for a meal.'

'Jewellery Quarter? Are you choosing a ring already?'

'No chance.' She grimaces, then stands and shucks her jacket on.

'Who is it, Jaz? Come on, anyone I know?'

'No.' Her lips curve in a quick embarrassed smile. She's lying.

'Jaz, seriously.' She won't look at me. 'Is it someone from work?'

She grabs her bag and throws it over her shoulder. Her cheeks flush. 'Honestly, it's just to shut him up, that's all.'

'Who?' Then the penny drops. All that flirting and teenage banter. I'm genuinely shocked. 'Matt?'

94

'Don't tell anyone at work.'

'No wonder you were sticking up for him.'

She laughs. 'Edie, I've tried every dating app going and met every weirdo in the West Midlands. You know my family; they've already given up hope on me meeting anyone.'

'But Matt? Seriously?'

She shrugs. 'I know. But it honestly feels like the only good thing I've got in my life sometimes is work. So any kind of date is better than going home to an empty flat.'

'All right, Jaz, it's your funeral. Just tell him if it was him who blabbed to Morris about me hanging around the department, he's dead.'

'You know Morris; he has ways of finding things out. But if it was Matt, I'll kill him myself. How's that?'

'It'll do.'

'I'd better go. Be kind to yourself, okay? And give me a call next week.'

She hugs me and winds her way through the pub. As soon as she is gone and I'm sitting on my own, her chair is pulled away by someone from a large, loud group nearby. I take my phone out. Still nothing from Harry. Frustrated, I tap the screen and call a taxi.

As the cab cuts past the converted factories of Digbeth, I lean my head against the window and watch the evening drinking crowds gathering at the bars. My head buzzes pleasantly from the wine, but the feeling is tempered by the lack of contact from Harry. He's been quiet all week and is now ignoring my texts. It wouldn't normally bother me, but after today it feels as though I'm being cut off on purpose. As the cab pulls along our row of terraces, I notice several lights on in our house. So he's home. I open the front door and can hear his voice coming from the kitchen in a one-sided conversation. He's using his telephone voice, and he's agitated. I ease the door shut, pull my shoes off and pad along the tiles of the hall to the kitchen. A shaft of light cuts across the hall as I stand near the gap. Harry is in the middle of an argument.

'Why have you done that, for God's sake?'

There is a long pause. His voice is sullen, resentful. He sounds like a morose adolescent. 'Well, what else am I supposed to think?'

He pauses again. I would hate to be eavesdropped on, but the decision has somehow made itself.

'I know, Dad,' Harry says eventually. 'But why keep it quiet?'

Dad? That explains it. My chest tightens and my mood hardens at the thought of James Creighton. A masochistic compulsion digs its claws into me and holds me there, listening. I have always hated being talked about, which ironically increases my sensitivity to whenever it's happening. Harry could be discussing anyone, but he's not. He's discussing me.

He makes an indistinct sound. Frustration? Annoyance? 'It's true, isn't it? I should have realised this a while ago.'

Should have realised what? His voice lifts again, indignant but also, in a subtle way, conceding. The beta male deferring to the alpha.

'She was right all along though, wasn't she?'

Long-held insecurities flood back once more. The feeling of being excluded, left out. Who was right, and about what? I can't tell if I'm being supported or let down by the man I want in my life forever, and that sense of isolation is now overwhelming.

'I'm not happy with this.' His voice is quieter. A long pause holds. 'Yeah, okay. You too. I'll see you soon.'

As he ends the call, I pad back to the front door, open it quietly and count to three, then slam it as if I've just come in. He appears in the doorway, a glass of wine in his hand.

'Hi.' He beams, as if everything is great with the world. 'I'll start dinner.'

I drop my work bag at the bottom of the stairs as he wanders over and hugs me.

'I heard voices as I came in,' I say, feigning nonchalance. 'Someone on the phone?'

'Yeah, Fergus, a mate from London. He's having a shit time with his girlfriend and wanted to vent. How was Jaz?' he asks.

'Fine.'

'Everything all right at work?' He is already on his way back to the kitchen.

'As good as it could be.' I follow him in, my thoughts tumbling over themselves. Should I call him out? Ask about the conversation? Demand to know what it was about? But I'm exhausted, done with other people's deception, done with their lies. Yes, the call may be completely innocent and, before all this happened, I'd have been prepared to give Harry the benefit of the doubt. But if so, why lie to me?

Before I reach the kitchen, I've made my mind up what I'm going to do. And it doesn't include Harry. He and his father can keep their little secrets.

The ones I care about are much closer to home.

17

Harry

Fuck! The alarm hasn't gone off. I've overslept.

It's my own stupid fault; the charger is temperamental, and I hadn't checked my phone was on charge last night. It must have died in the middle of the night and is now a useless lump of metal. At least the clock radio Edie wakes up to every morning is reliable. She still uses it because it was a teenage present from her mother, but I can't stand its cheap, tinny noise. I hate it even more now, as its red digits spell out the time: 8:04. Swearing under my breath, I wiggle the charger and wait for the percentage to creep up, sorting through my day, scanning my memory for important appointments. Luckily, I have nothing on until an MDT meeting at ten. By the time I've showered, the phone is on eight per cent, so I dress with it wedged between my ear and shoulder as I tell work I'm running late, then I head downstairs.

Halfway down, I get that empty house vibe. It's obvious that Edie has already left for work, and there's a quick stab of irritation that she didn't wake me. In the kitchen, my eyes scan the untidy pile of last night's washing-up at the sink before finally resting on the table. That's when I see the note, laid in front of a small vase of wilting flowers, which Edie bought a week ago, before all this began. As I stare at the note, a vague sense of unease brushes my neck with icy fingers. She's upset at what's happened, but she wouldn't do *that*, surely? But I've assessed too many suicidal people to ignore the morbid thought that springs into my mind, uninvited. No, there is no way she would. She's too stubborn, for one thing. I scan the hastily written page, and the thought evaporates in the first line. *Harry, I need time to think.* I read on; the rest is brief and to the point. She's leaving for a few days to clear her head. It's not my fault, apparently. This whole thing has come as a shock and she needs space. She doesn't elaborate. The last few lines are blunt, not like her at all.

Don't phone me, I won't answer.

My thoughts drift back to last night, replaying everything. What is going on in her mind she's not sharing with me? You believe you know someone, convince yourself they've let you in, then you're stumbling around in the dark again. She was quiet yesterday, but then I suppose we've both been quiet for days. Her mother admitting herself to Claydon Manor rocked her; that much was obvious. Jenny's harsh whisper comes back to me. *It will ruin yours too.* What did she mean? I can understand how thin the armour that stops this trauma shredding their lives is, and I can understand why they don't face it head on. But *ruined*? It's too final, too dramatic. We all hide from ourselves to different degrees; that's part of being an adult. If we felt every childhood insult and agony with the same intensity of the original, we would all need locking away. Instead, we remember fragments of the past, our memories nothing but faded replays, ghosts, inventions, worn-out copies. And I know, because I hide my array of neuroses and anxieties in exactly the same way. Why else are us psychiatrists drawn to explore the human psyche in the first place, if not from being as damaged as the rest?

I put the letter back down on the table. Did she overhear the conversation with my father last night? If so, she would have seen through my lie about Fergus as soon as it tumbled out. She won't realise I was lying to protect her. The relationship between sons and fathers forms the most complicated chapter in the textbook, as adversaries in the most instinctive and violent part of the Oedipal complex. I wish he could sense my contempt every time he interferes in my life. It would be bad enough if Edie realised it was him and that I'd lied to her, but it would be ten times worse if she knew what he'd said. He even reacted as though it had accidentally slipped out of his mouth, but once it was there it hung between us and could not be unsaid. The revelation that set my incredulous heart pounding is here for good, and I have to find a way of dealing with it. Edie's sense of trust must be fragile enough already.

If I don't play this carefully, it will shatter forever.

The MDT meeting is to discuss a care plan for Josh Bellmore, who is still struggling to accept his diagnosis. When I hear myself saying that a patient has trouble accepting a condition, I always question my approach to these situations. I get caught up in the language of our profession, buying into those words we use so often they've lost meaning. Acceptance, denial, medication, management, control. We sit there, calm and rational, but any of us would be just like Josh if we'd watched the scenery of our lives collapsing around us like he had. The usual suspects are at the table; Naomi Bagley, the lead psychiatric nurse on the unit, sits next to clinical psychologist John Casement, an old-school Freudian who dutifully fights the corner for the talking cure. Then there is a social worker, an occupational therapist and the pharmacist, Gaia Bakshi, a tired-looking woman who smiles approvingly as I summarise the powerful antipsychotics we've been giving to Josh. I represent the medical side of the team, the front line of these emergency cases.

As the talk continues, and the care plan that will structure Josh's life for the next few months gets built, my attention drifts back to the note Edie left. A plan has been forming as the voices in the meeting become a monotone hum. As soon as the meeting ends, I make my excuses to leave. The secure unit is a modern, red-brick block, bolted on to the main Victorian building where our offices are, but there is no direct access between the unit and the administrative floors. This suits me fine; I don't want to go through the main offices anyway, in case I meet Amy Wilson. Ever since Edie began sessions with her, I've made a point of having as little to do with Amy as possible to avoid any accusations of conflict of interest. It's even more awkward since Edie stormed out on her. I skirt the edge of the building and cross a patch of scrubby grass onto the main car park of the hospital, pulling my lanyard out as I head towards the ambulance entrance.

Going through the Emergency Department is the quickest route to ICU and theatres, although there's always the obstacle course of trolleys and patients to negotiate. The lift to the ICU is behind the ED, and I bump into Matt Phillips coming out, a white coat over his scrubs, cigarette packet in hand.

'Hi, it's Matt, right?' I ask. 'Have you got a minute?'

He frowns briefly, obviously in a hurry, then recognises me. 'Oh yeah. Harry. How's things? I haven't seen you for ages.'

'Yeah, I'm good. This is a weird thing to have to ask, but has Edie taken some time off work?' I look at my phone and shrug. 'I can't actually get hold of her right now.'

His round face drops, and a flicker of confusion flits across it. Or is it panic? He puffs his cheeks and runs his fingers across his hair. 'You don't know what's happened?'

'No, I haven't had a chance to talk to her since yesterday.'

He pauses. 'Mate, she's been put on sick leave for a few weeks. You know, because… well, you know.'

He's floundering, so I take pity on him. 'Right, I understand. Whose decision was that?'

'Richard Morris, I imagine.'

'Okay. Thanks, Matt. I'll catch up with her later.'

He nods and brushes past, glad to escape the awkwardness. Once he has disappeared down the corridor and I'm alone, I tap my phone screen. Six months ago, I'd bought Edie a brand-new iPhone for her birthday. The cost was eye-watering, so before I'd given it to her I'd downloaded the Find My app in case it was stolen, and paired it with my phone. I hadn't mentioned it to her at the time; it didn't seem important. Now it feels like the best decision I've made in months. I open the app and the map springs up. Edie's smiling face appears as a tiny round icon. She is approaching Bristol on the M5, moving towards the coast. Heading back to the village where Samuel Cox took her.

But what happens when she discovers what's waiting there? What if her mother's whispered warning is true? She'll need someone with her, someone to pick up the pieces. And after what my father admitted last night, there's another reason I'm going to have to follow her. I need to speak to her.

Bad news should always be delivered in person.

18

Edie

May 15th 2004

It's going to take some planning, but I know the date now. I've booked three weeks annual leave starting 20th June. Three weeks, so no one will miss me for a while. I told them I'm going to stay with some relatives. It clearly didn't show in my expression that I'm leaving for good, that I'm done with the whole fucking thing. I know now that this is the right thing to do, and I'm going to follow it through, no matter how it ends. If there's any justice in the world, the truth will come to light one day. I don't care how much I suffer for her, I've got to do something. My manager Doug had smiled behind his thick, grey walrus moustache, patted my arm. To be honest, mate, he said, we were going to tell you to have some time off anyway. He managed a sympathetic frown. We're worried about you.

I knew what he meant, I understood the implication. I'd come in the previous morning hungover and stinking of booze. Not for the first time, either. It was always the same pattern, I'd just want to blot things out, but then once you start drinking you lose track of time. I have driven myself crazy thinking of what I could have done differently, how this could have turned out better. I know I'm to blame, and guilt is a hard thing to erase from your mind. So I needed a little help from alcohol to get on top of it. In the last couple of years, I'd got into the habit of always making sure there was a bottle in the house – always hidden, because otherwise Mel would find it and tip it down the sink, thinking she was helping me. I don't know why I've put her through this for so long, I should have done the right thing months ago and just left her.

Doug signed the leave sheet as I watched. He might think he's getting rid of me for a while to sort my head out. That I'll be back soon. Only I know that, once I leave his office today, we'll never see each other again.

May 22nd 2004

I'll take her back there. I'll take her where no one will find us.

Today I sat and watched the house. It is a Saturday, so I could wait all morning. I've got my place, where the car is out of sight. I can sit here and see when they come and go. I can watch him put his golf clubs in the boot of that BMW of his, with those personalised number plates. X3 MAC, Michael Alan Carter. You think you're untouchable, but your days are numbered, you smug bastard.

You might have fooled everyone else, but I know what you've been doing.

I've been watching them every Saturday, so I know what their routine is. They are all creatures of habit, I know that already. I probably know his family better than he does. If only he realised. I'm cutting back on the drinking. I have to take this seriously now, it's given me a purpose. Mel thinks I'm turning a corner, she's happy for me, I get the feeling she thinks there is a chance for us, but she's wrong. I'm too far gone, there is too much pain for me ever to be right again. I told her last night that she should leave me but she says she loves me. More guilt. Now I know even more clearly what I've done, the depth of my betrayal. But I don't need self-pity, I need redemption.

He leaves at nine-thirty. At ten, her mother leaves the house to go to the shops. E is not with her. Her mother walks along the street a few yards, stops to talk to a neighbour. She is a beautiful woman, E looks a lot like her. It's an overcast day, but she has sunglasses on. Why? Maybe he hurts her too, punishes her like he punishes E. I know I'm not imagining the guilty air she carries; perhaps she thinks she deserves it. Does she know what's happening to her daughter, like I think she does? Is it fear behind those glasses too, or helplessness?

It won't be long now.

I could come and take you today, you must be in the house, I arrived at this spot at seven, half-hidden behind the block of garages across the road. You are in there. Shall I come and get you now? Have you had enough? Can you put up with just a few weeks more?

I wait, and I watch. I time the visit to the shops, when he gets back from golf. I will be here next Saturday to do the same thing again.

I can't prove anything, but I know what your fear means, E. He might be able to hide it from everyone else, but not from me. I promise you, it won't be long.

It won't be long.

A shadow falls across the page as a man sits opposite me, and I'm thrust back into the noise of the Costa at Sedgemoor services. Disorientated, I cover the journal with my hand. The man is suited and in his mid-fifties, with wispy grey hair and glasses. He stirs his coffee with an irritating tinkle of spoon against cup.

'I hope you don't mind me joining you?' he asks, waving his arm at the busy tables. 'There didn't seem to be any other chairs.'

'No, it's fine.'

He continues to smile at me, radiating the cloying vibe of a conversation-starved salesman. The last thing I want to do is make small talk, so I keep my eyes down, flicking through the journal until he gets the message and begins studying his phone.

Until today, the diary had been in the drawer next to my bed, untouched for days. I'd begun to understand why Melanie Cox only read snatches of it, and how obsessive Cox was in the months before the abduction. There is no filter between us as I read, and I'm watching a mind unravel in slow, horrible detail. But where is the predator the papers described? Where is the abuser lurking in those hastily written pages? All I've found is desperation, helplessness, irrationality, as he shifts the blame for what he did to my father.

My father. All I get when I visualise him is an unfamiliar man grinning from old photos. A stranger smiling in holiday snaps; tall, dark-haired, handsome in a stocky way. But he won't coalesce into a living, moving person. There is always a vacancy when I think of my parents when they were young, which sometimes feels like it existed from the moment I was born. My earliest sensations are of no one being there. Of two blank mother- and father-shaped spaces. As I got older, I never even grieved properly for the void that was left. I know he died suddenly because that's what I was told. *His heart gave out*, was the way my mother phrased it. Now I know the technical term. Myocardial infarction. Michael Carter was, and forever has been, part of my twilight world. Samuel Cox blamed him, hated him. But diaries lie, don't they? Convicted kidnappers and abusers lie. They build excuses, reasons.

The picture painted of Cox by the newspaper reports showed a very different person to the one I'm reading about in the diary. There was a press embargo on many of the details, but they hinted darkly at what he did, how brazen the abduction was, how terrible the abuse must have been. They made it clear the abuse was sexual, but there were no details made public of course. My mother and I were kept out of it, but they went to town on Cox, building a picture of a monster. I force my memory to provide details of the abduction, but it won't. All I have access to are vague scenes from some detached, barely remembered story. Was I screaming in the back seat as I was driven away? Were there tears on my cheeks? If so, where has the fear of this man gone now? I would remember fear, wouldn't I? I should be terrified of retracing this journey, yet I'm not.

Day by day the net had closed around him, the reports said. In the end, it had taken a dog walker on the coastal path to spot him with me, follow him, and finally alert the police to his exact location. In the bedroom of a cottage in a village near Watchet, on the morning of 12 August 2004, it ended. When I close my eyes, I can almost hear the echo of loud voices, the banging on the door, see a ghost of the blue police lights through the curtains. Just traces of the time he had me, scenes from a film you used to know well but are now forgotten. Sometimes, as I read page after page of lurid reporting, I can nearly touch how I must have felt in those interview rooms amongst the specially trained officers. Faceless and nameless, embodiments of the emptiness and vulnerability that floods over me whenever I try to remember what it felt like as a child.

According to the reports, Samuel Cox had confessed so there was no reason to drag such a young girl through the courts. Another lost memory I'm spared. But they'd found psychological 'evidence' of abuse, whatever that meant. There were details deemed to show too much knowledge for someone of eight to have invented, too specific to be fabricated. A child psychologist had been wheeled out to testify and claimed the residual trauma was the worst he'd ever dealt with. The most damaged child of his career, he'd said, as if there should be some prize for it. Nice to have your abnormality confirmed. This was all in the papers. Damaged, what a lazy word. What exactly do they mean by that? And what do they ever do afterwards to repair such damage? The reports had carried the pictures of the angry men and women banging the sides of the blue van as it pulled away, with its small, high windows, behind which Samuel Cox was hiding. I could imagine him cowering inside. Whatever he felt at that moment was nothing compared to what he would suffer in prison.

Nearly twenty years spent looking over his shoulder, waiting for the next blow. Taunts, insults, threats. Violence. No one would have cared; it was nothing less than he deserved. Yet none of the malice and evil they accused him of is there in the neat lines of his journal. Nothing of the evil they described was there when I looked at him in ICU.

I drop the diary back in my bag. How close to Cox's real voice is the one that speaks from the pages? If he woke from his anaesthetic, would his voice be the same as I imagine it? If a landscape holds memories, then I'm getting closer. As the miles had passed, I'd questioned why I was coming back here, but the answer is obvious if I admit it to myself. To discover the truth. To be whole again. And in the meantime I have Samuel Cox's voice for company, talking to me. Just as he did then.

It won't be long.

19

Samuel Cox

The ventilator hisses, marking the passing of his life, the life he thought would already be over. The drifting is interminable. Purgatory. He had heard of anaesthetic awareness, the state of existing and not existing at the same time, caught in between sleep and wakefulness. Now it is happening to him. How long has it been? Voices come and go, thoughts drift in and out, taking the shape of dreams or nightmares. But the worst of it is over. There can be no more of the guilt that has built up over the years, driving him insane, making him care so little for his life that he began hoping to be killed in prison. He didn't even fight back when they came for him, time after time.

But now it's done. After two years of probation; days of drifting, unemployment, endless drinking. Cheap, gut-rot alcohol. Thinking about her. And now she has seen the message he brought. She will understand the pain and the sacrifice he went through to get the message to her. She will know that he wasn't to blame. He was trapped in a compulsion, obsessed with her. He wasn't rational.

He thought he would only survive for a few hours after the tablets; that was all he needed. He had been so careful to calculate the dose. Enough to kill him slowly. Just enough amitriptyline to get him admitted to ICU long enough for her to see his message. He had taken his age into account, his weight, his liver function. He had saved for private blood tests, and had not cared when many of the markers came back as abnormal. The clinic recommended he see his doctor immediately, unaware of his real motives. He could have faced her, waited for her after work, but that would mean breaking his parole terms and going back to prison. It wasn't the *right* thing to do. He could have sent her a letter, but that was too impersonal.

This way makes sense to him. This way, they will all know how he really feels. This is repentance for everyone he hurt. Atonement.

Except he is still alive. He had got it wrong, and now he waits.

Do you understand yet, Edie? Will you remember me the way I want to be remembered? Do you still remember the truth?

Dark, broken images come and go. Replays of the sentencing, of those first few years in prison. The confession, the brief trial, the stony-faced police officers who looked at him as though they would happily kill him themselves if they had a chance.

Voices, drifting again. He hears the nurse who has looked after him the most. She jokes and laughs sometimes; he pictures her smiling often. He sometimes hears the name. Jaz.

She is with him now; he can hear her talking to someone else, distant.

'Okay, I'll be there in a minute. I'm just measuring this guy's urine output.'

'It's getting better.'

'What? He's coming to see him? Okay, I'll be there now. I don't want to be around when Morris is here anyway, the guy gives me the creeps.'

Morris, the doctor. The one who was here when he first came in. It may have been months ago, it may have been hours. Under sedation, time doesn't matter. Then more voices, they are next to him. He recognises Morris's voice; the other is indistinct, quiet.

'Yes, this is the fellow. He was the one who took Doctor Carter when she was a child.'

The other voice speaks. Male. Clipped like Morris. He cannot hear what is said. Then Morris again.

'Absolutely. We have tried to get her to talk this through rationally, but she seems intent on dealing with things her own way.'

He hears the other voice, indistinct.

'Yes, she is an excellent doctor. But I think you are right. We need to manage her.'

Indistinct again.

'Amy and I agree. This needs to be handled carefully.'

Murmurs, closer. 'Keep me informed, Richard, would you? I don't think things are quite as they seem with this fellow.'

'Of course.'

'I must get back. I'm speaking at three.'

Then silence again, except for the constant ventilator, the gentle beeps of the machine, the occasional soft whirr of an infusion pump.

Death does not frighten him. But perhaps he will wake and she will be there.

He can tell her everything. He feels as protective as he did all those years ago.

He still loves her now as he did then. Loved her *too* much, perhaps. No one understood her except him.

The men were talking about her. Be careful, Edie.

He drifts. Maybe everything happens for a reason. Maybe he will live. He will wake up, and he will finally see her again. Talk to her.

And then she will know the truth.

20

Edie

The A39 carries a steady flow of traffic through the village of Stowell, although no one seems to stop there. Yesterday the weather had turned as I came past Bridgwater, and by the time I reached the village a slow, steady drizzle had begun falling. As the rain darkened the grey stone of the houses, a bleak mood had settled on me as I drove around the narrow streets, recognising nothing. This is the place the papers said he came, but my memory is as uncooperative as always. Nothing fits as I hoped it would. Somewhere in this village, he had rented the cottage where we'd remained for the two weeks it took them to track us down. Once he had collected the keys, telling the owner he was here with his daughter, we were alone. He had me all to himself for two weeks, the papers said, implying there was nothing to stop him doing whatever he wanted. The headlines managed to be graphic and suggestive without giving details. *Innocence Lost. The Captive of a Fiend. A Fortnight in Hell.* But we were spotted on a local cliff path, by someone who recognised him from the papers. The reports never explained why, if I was his unwilling prisoner, we went for walks together. If I was so traumatised then, why didn't I run?

Finally frustrated as evening fell, I stopped driving and pulled in at the local village pub. When I asked if he had a room to let, the landlord looked pointedly around the almost empty, earthy-smelling saloon bar.

'Yes, love,' he said rolling his eyes, 'I think I can squeeze you in.'

He was around sixty, and my first instinct as a doctor was to tell him to ask his GP for statins. Red-faced and round-bellied, solid in a way only men who have been eating and drinking to excess for decades can be, he prowled the bar with the sway of a large animal.

'Have you been here long?' I asked, as he passed me the room key.

He nodded, wiping the gouged, dull wooden bar top. 'Since ninety-six. Long enough to be working bloody pub hours, eh?' He scanned the few customers he had, most of whom were nursing a lonely drink. 'Time for me to retire maybe?'

Behind the cynicism, his smile was genuine and easy, and it struck me that, even though it seemed to be slowly killing him, there was no other profession he'd rather be doing. My hand reached into my bag for the photo, then paused. As I held the picture, I felt weary of it all, and the urge to drop the room key on the bar and leave this whole pointless pilgrimage behind overwhelmed me. In the end, the landlord made the decision for me.

'What's that?' he asked, nodding at the photo.

Still hesitant, I held it out. 'It's a bit of a long shot. But do you recognise either of these girls? Or the bay where this was taken?'

He glanced at the photo, then at me. Shutting one eye like he was taking aim, he studied it again. He pointed a sausage-sized, stubby finger. 'Seeing as you're in the photo, how come you don't remember yourself? That *is* you, isn't it?'

I was too tired to explain. 'Yeah. But I just don't remember much about it.'

'Is that other girl your sister?'

I'd stared at the other young girl, her arm draped over my shoulder. I studied her straight white smile, her elfin bones. I thought of my mother's writing. *Edie and Sophie.* The landlord was right: we could be sisters. Looking at Sophie's face was like trying to recall a forgotten melody, a once-loved tune that has slipped from your mind. 'I don't know. I've come here to try to find out.'

'Sorry, love. I've never seen either her or that bay before. But then, there are dozens of beaches like that along this part of the coast. Could be anywhere.'

I thanked him and went to my room, feeling more alone than ever, as if the threads holding together my sense of self were as thin as cotton. The room was neat and clean but as tired and outdated as the rest of the pub. I lay on the floral duvet of the single bed and closed my eyes, dropping into a troubled sleep as the rain tapped the window.

Later, after I'd eaten a bland plate of fish and chips with peas like bullets, I tried the photo on locals, getting nothing but pitying glances and slow shakes of the head. Some barely looked at it. I'd had enough for the day. None of the memories I'd tried to trigger in people by coming here had materialised. No one knew anything. I headed back up the creaking stairs to my room, the fish and chips already repeating on me.

Next morning, sitting out in the small, walled back garden with a strong coffee, as the last clouds disperse and the sky lightens, I feel ready to try again. This time I'm going on foot; to walk the village, every street and alleyway, to recreate everything and see what comes, no matter how painful. To drag myself back into the past on my own terms. I check my phone. Nothing from Harry. The signal flickers from one bar to no service; I don't even know if I'm reachable here.

Stowell is on a low hill; half the village winds down towards the coast a mile away, while the rest is on a series of inclines, each having a better elevation and view than the ones below it. Several of the larger houses on the highest incline look empty, although the place doesn't seem affluent enough to attract second homeowners. As I meander my way down from the top, the morning sun hits the slate-coloured stone and lights the flowers and shrubs in the gardens. This place could be pretty in summer with its run-down charm. As I walk, I finally pin down what has been bothering me since I arrived. I've felt no apprehension here. No dread or worry. Whatever sensations are being evoked by the village where Samuel Cox hid out for two weeks, fear isn't one of them. Melancholy, perhaps. Wistfulness, a sense of something lost. But not pain. I turn a corner at the end of a small street where the fields begin, dropping down towards the main road. The sea glitters dark green in the distance. I turn into a narrow road with a sign saying *No Vehicle Access*.

Then I'm there.

The cottage is on the corner, alone, invisible from the road, surrounded by a low wall and gardens. The nearest neighbour is thirty yards away, where the winding street leads back towards the village. The second-storey windows are blank, catching the sky and reflecting its late spring blue. The frames of the windows are wood, painted a dark green against the lighter stonework. The front door is not the same as it was then. Modern, sturdy oak stands where there used to be an old half-and-half stable door. The front garden has had a patio laid, someone has added a small extension to the back where the kitchen used to be. I walk to the front gate and rest my hand on it, easing it open. The wood feels rough under my hand.

It's the place. This is where we came.

The power of the recollection is so strong it takes me a moment to remember I'm an adult again, seeing everything from an adult's perspective. This is exactly as I imagined it, just as I knew it would be.

'Can I help you, young lady?'

The front door has opened, and a woman in her late sixties is looking at me, a puzzled smile on her face as I stand halfway inside her gate, one hand still resting on it. My heart is hammering, my breath is pulling.

'Oh, I'm sorry,' I manage.

'Don't apologise. Can I help you at all?'

I squint past the woman into the house beyond; the brightness of the morning obscures the interior, but I know I would recognise every corner and wall, the stairs and the layout. I know the back garden even though I can't see it. It is not a memory as much as a pure feeling, as though I'm seeing the reality behind a perfect, faultless description of the place. But there is one thing I'm finally certain of as I look at the house. It is a place of safety. Nothing bad took place here.

'No, I'm fine. Sorry.' I turn to leave, but I'm caught by the centripetal force of the recollection. 'Actually, I just wanted to ask you some questions about the house.'

'Well, don't stand in the garden; come inside for a moment.'

'No,' I say, too fast. 'No, thanks.'

'I can't talk to you from the gate.' She smiles. 'Come on, don't be shy.'

I walk up the path towards the front door, following in his steps twenty years earlier, my heart trying to escape from my chest. Then I'm at the door. The woman steps aside to let me in and without thinking I've crossed the threshold. The stairs are where I expected them to be; three steps to a small landing, a ninety-degree angle to the upstairs. The balustrade is the same but painted white instead of varnished wood. The door to the kitchen is open and I can see the long, wooden breakfast bar. We sat there and ate together each morning. Beyond is sunlight through windows, and that's where the garden is, where we sat outside on sunny days. I'm calmer, my pulse is slowing. Standing in this hallway I don't feel the cold tattered remnants of fear or terror, but safety. Friendship. Love, even.

I'm now becoming more certain of one thing, that perhaps I alone in the whole world know. Samuel Cox is innocent. I don't know what he wants forgiveness for, but it's not for abusing me.

'Can I ask how long you've lived here for?' I don't even realise I've spoken until I hear the woman's voice in reply.

'A while. Are you doing a survey?'

'No…' I hesitate. I'm thrust back into the present, my mind scrabbling for excuses to be here. 'I was just wondering about the area. We're thinking of moving down this way.'

'We've been here for ten years,' she replies. 'Moved down from Bristol. I'd recommend it. It's a lovely village.'

'Do you know who had the house before?'

'No, my dear. I think the previous owner died. Anyway, it was vacant when we moved in.'

I mumble my thanks and, with one last look at the hallway, turn back down the path and towards the village. I try to consciously put myself back in the past, to be that child who was carried through the door of the cottage twenty years ago. But nothing else will come back other than what I've seen and felt; the place continues to be a tumbledown, sun-washed Somerset village, and I am back to being a tourist who is looking at it through fresh eyes. But the certainty and the strength of how I felt in that hallway remain.

I make my way towards the road, so I can cross to the coastal side of the village. On the opposite side is the pub. There are only three cars in the car park at this time of the morning. My beaten-up Renault, a blue BMW... and as I cross the road, I can see the third one more clearly.

An old black Audi, a familiar number plate.

Harry.

21

Harry

Across the saloon bar, her eyes are boring into me with a silent, furious question. *What are you doing here?* I don't know why I was expecting anything else; I should have realised how this must look. She already feels scrutinised, controlled. But she doesn't know what I know yet, and I'm still trying to think of a way of telling her. Things like this make me realise what a coward I am, how much I dodge conflict. I could have called her and told her yesterday, but I convinced myself it should be done face to face. Now I'm here and I'm still not ready. She stands in the pub doorway, staring at me while I stir my coffee. For all my good intentions, embarrassment washes over me as she approaches.

'Edie, let me explain.'

She sits down. Nobody in the bar notices the tension. 'How did you know I was here?'

'Come on, have a coffee first.'

'I don't want a coffee. How did you find me?'

I lay my phone on the table, face-up. She studies the two icons on the map, tiny round faces. Hers and mine. 'Your new phone, Edes. I downloaded Find My. It was supposed to be a security thing, not for... this.'

She glares at me, her green eyes flashing. 'I'm surprised you didn't bring Morris, Wilson and your parents along.'

'I'm sorry, but I couldn't just ignore you, could I?'

She pushes my phone away and shakes her head, lips pinched. 'I can't believe you did this, Harry. This isn't some twisted game of hide and seek.'

117

'Look, I want to help you. We might not always agree on things, but I'm not going to just sit back and let you do this alone.'

'It's not up to you though, is it?' She picks at the scab on her thumb again. I hold her hand to stop her, but she draws it away. 'And anyway, stop playing innocent.'

My stomach clenches. 'What are you on about?'

'It wasn't Fergus on the phone last night, was it? It wasn't a London friend, or some mate from school, or work telling you how wonderful you are, so cut the excuses.'

How much did she hear? Despite what my father had told me about his new job – the bombshell that made me lie to Edie about the call – he denied every accusation I put to him about why he took it. He has this way of turning things around. He was playing it cool as he always does, twisting the focus back onto me again, so I ended up feeling like a wilful child. He manoeuvres me, *manages* me, leaving me with a tight, grinding sense of injustice, which can sometimes last for days. But where did Edie come in on the conversation? How much of its meaning did she work out? God, no wonder she came here on her own to get away from us all. I look at the turmoil in her eyes, the repetitive, nervous picking of her thumbnail, and hate myself for not having the courage yet to admit why I'm here.

'I'm sorry. I should have told you who it was on the phone. But I know how much you mistrust him.'

'But you won't have a bad word said.' She finds anything else in the bar to focus other than me. 'You take his side every time. The dinner party was the first time I've ever seen you criticise him.'

I fall silent. She's right, most of my rebellion has always been internal. In the two years we've known each other, I can't remember taking her side in any meaningful way against my family. When my father, icily polite but unbearably superior, would make her feel small, I'd tell her she was imagining it. Nicky's invite to the party was not *their* fault, it was Edie's problem for misinterpreting it. On almost every occasion, I've given my parents a free pass to act like snobs. But I know myself well, better than I share with others, even Edie. And while I may have seemed a bit spineless, even to get this far is an act of determination. If Edie was anyone else, we wouldn't have lasted this long. With anyone else, my father's disapproval would have worn me down long ago.

'I'm sorry,' I say eventually, realising she has been watching me closely. 'I know I should have supported you against them more. But I do love you, Edie. I don't think you realise how much.'

The barman is at our end of the bar, standing right behind us, polishing glasses. Neither of us had noticed him; for a man of his size he moves surprisingly quietly. Edie glances at him; he catches her look and smiles, not understanding we want to be left alone. Something bugs me about his lack of awareness. I stand and lean towards him.

'Excuse me, a bit of privacy would be nice.'

'Sorry mate, I…' He tails off.

'Harry?' Edie glances at the barman. 'Sorry.'

The barman gives me a dirty look and ambles away as I sit down. Why did I snap at him? It's not his fault I don't know how to tell Edie what my father said. 'Edie, I'm sorry. I don't know why I reacted.'

'What's got into you?'

'I said I was sorry.'

After a moment, she leans forward, my apology finally accepted. 'Listen, Harry, seeing you isn't the first shock of the morning.'

'How do you mean?'

'I've found the cottage where he took me.'

'So you've remembered what happened here?'

She sighs. 'Not exactly, not everything. But I know it's the place.'

'And are you okay?' I take her hand. Her head has dropped, and a thick strand of dark hair has fallen across her face.

'Yeah. But I wasn't scared. Why is that?' I'm expecting emotion, but when she looks up her eyes are dry, her expression flat. 'Harry, he wasn't the monster they think he is.'

'Oh Edes, you just want what he did to go away, that's all. Dissociation and repression are powerful coping mechanisms, and denial is just as strong too. But you're probably sick of being told that.'

'Yet again, everyone knows what's best except me.'

'I didn't mean it like that.' A blast of cool air comes through the pub as the door opens and a customer comes in. The barman moves to the end of the bar to serve him and the two men start talking. 'Look, how about we go for a drive along the coast?'

'I don't know, Harry. Why? This is something I want to do alone.'

'Give me that photo a minute,' I ask. I want to show her that I'm here to help. That I'm on her side. She pulls the crumpled photo out of her pocket and lays it on the table. I scan the coastline behind the two girls and point to the bay. 'Because if you want to remember, we need to find where this was taken.'

We've pulled into every small bay for miles. Wherever the road dips down to the sea, we've followed it. Edie has been checking the photograph as I drive, but it's me who has been reading the topography of the coastline, keeping one eye on the road as I crane my neck to see over distant hedgerows and trees. At this time of year, the Bristol Channel is an estuarial green brown, nothing like the leaden blue of the sea behind the two girls in the photo, and I'm starting to regret my idea. We're almost certainly wasting our time, but, having been the one to suggest it, I can't help but keep going. As we approach Doniford, I pull into a small side road leading towards the sea. This must be the tenth at least. Ahead is a sign, pointing the way to a caravan site. Denham Farm. Underneath in faded yellow are the words *Beach Access*.

'Let's try here.' I stop, and Edie holds the photo out, contrasting it to the scenery. I lean over to look. 'That outcrop over there looks a bit like the one behind you and Sophie.'

'Harry, look at the sea. It's a different colour completely.'

'The photo is over twenty years old, Edes. The light is different, that's all.'

'You're the one who wanted to stalk me all the way here, so promise this will be the last one then? I'm not going to remember anything.'

'You remembered the cottage.'

'I know, but that was something specific. This is just coastline.'

'Okay, last one.'

The car winds through a dappled wood, the road falling gradually down as the landscape slopes towards the coast. Through gaps in the trees we catch glimpses of the sea, then we are passing static caravans, hidden away in jumbled plots. The road widens out into a small, gravel car park, with a sign to the clubhouse and one to the beach. The walk down is steep, winding down a cliff fifty feet above a wide sweeping bay. To the far left, the sails of the holiday camp at Minehead shine white, gleaming in the distance. To the right, the coast fades into obscurity, in a series of small bays and headlands, finally meeting the horizon. Although clouds are gathering above the headland, the day is still bright and clear and I can make out the coast of South Wales at the edge of my vision.

Edie is walking a few steps behind, looking along the coast, as I alternately study the photograph and the small bay in front of us. As we get closer to the stones and rocks below, a steadily increasing buzz of anticipation courses through me. She was wrong to write this place off so quickly. The tide is out, and, beyond the twenty yards of rocks and stones that lie at the foot of the cliff, the sand is brown and fine. Where it has dried it has a colour like dark honey, and further out the wet flats are like polished oak. The waves lap onto the beach in small, gentle undulations.

At the sight of the headland to the left, my heart trips faster.

It could be.

Edie is several steps behind me on the rocks now as I hold the photograph up towards the far headland, turning it so I can make comparisons. My voice has to carry some distance to her on the breeze, and I hear it rise and fall with a blend of excitement and fear.

'Edie. Look.'

She jogs to catch up with me, her chin against my neck as she stands on tiptoe to look over my shoulder. Behind the two girls in the photograph, the coastline is identical. In the near distance there is a waterfall at the end of the headland. I let my eyes drift beyond the photograph to the cliffs ahead of us. The sun catches the water in precisely the same way, the waterfall is the same. The headland has the same contours, even down to the trees leaning precariously at the edge. We are standing almost precisely where the photograph was taken all those years ago. But there is something else too. This is the first time I've looked at the photo this closely, the first time I've examined it like this. The faces of the two girls are happy, they're smiling, their eyes hidden behind the star-shaped sunglasses. But there's something there I hadn't noticed before. A reflection.

'Edie, look at Sophie's sunglasses.'

Edie studies the photograph. She lays it down on a large rock, holds it with one hand and takes her phone out, getting the camera as close as she can, adjusting the focus until the girl's face fills the frame. I squat next to her and we shade our eyes as we examine Sophie's image. With two fingers, Edie zooms in, closer and closer. The glasses get larger, the image gets clearer.

In her sunglasses is a figure. A tiny reflection of the person who took the photograph.

The enlarged image is grainy, but visible.

'Take a photograph and clarify it,' I hiss. 'There'll be a studio function on your phone. You can sharpen the image.'

Edie hits some buttons, her hands shaking. Image. Sharpen. Maximum. We shade our eyes again and look at the result.

Mirrored in Sophie's sunglasses is the photograph taker, holding the camera low, near his chest. I have to squint to make the image coalesce in front of my eyes. Then I see him, I know him. The blurry face of the man taking this smiling holiday photograph of Edie and Sophie is visible. He is recognisable from the images in the paper. The date on the back said July 2003. This photograph was taken less than a year before he abducted her. So much for him being a random stalker.

But they say it's always someone the victim knows.

The man holding the camera is Samuel Cox.

22

Edie

I remember the day felt like the hottest of the year, the warmest of my life.

We ran in and out of the sea to cool down. I was more confident to begin with, but she got braver once we became wet and got used to the gentle push and pull of the waves. The sand seemed to stretch forever where the tide had gone out, leaving a shiny brown playground with small popping bubbles where air was escaping. The suntan lotion on my skin was slick, and streaky where the sea had mixed with it. We ran from where the rocks started to where the waves were washing the shore, our wet feet slapping on the sand, our hair flying, glancing at each other and screaming with laughter as we both tried to be the first to splash into the shallows. Our knees lifted higher and higher, pumping like pistons as we ran deeper and further, and then there was a scream and a spray of foam. Of the two of us, I can't remember who the first one in was, but I remember us diving deep under the water, again and again.

Where's Edie? he called from the shore. I waved back. *We're okay.*

I sometimes stayed under for ages to get his attention, and when I resurfaced we would giggle as we watched him shake his head as he stood by the line of surf.

That summer was made up of days, not just moments. The day was one of many but is the only one that comes back in such vivid colours. We got to the beach mid-morning, when the sun was halfway up the sky, rising above the brown and green cliffs to our right, silhouetting the single trees dotting the coastline, as small and thin as toothpicks in the distance. Where the sand began, he set the windbreak up, those broad stripes of primary colours that had no wind to protect us from, as the day was warm and still. Instead it was our changing room, a place to get into swimsuits, wrapped in towels, a place to leave all of our beach toys for the day. The ball, the small dinghy, the kite that would lie still and dry on the sand. All were piled behind the rectangles of coloured cotton, one of only a few on the beach. It was a quiet, almost undiscovered bay, where no crowds came, even in the summer.

He looked similar then, but he was a different person, in the sense features never change but perspective does. Young, with sideburns, short, tousled hair. It was dark and roughed by the seawater that had dried in it after he chased us both into the sea and splashed around. His eyes seemed an impossibly light green to me, maybe because the sun was shining so brightly on the water. He would smile, but to me the smile felt troubled and broken somehow, as if I had some deeper access to empathy as a child, some increased sensitivity in the mirror neurons. He was happy, yes, but he was also absent in a way I couldn't understand. He would play for a while, lifting us onto his shoulder and throwing us into the water. Then we would run back for him to do it all over again. It's strange how the emotions of the day are as new to me again now as the colours are, or the smell of the sea, the coconut of the sunscreen, and my toes sinking in the sand.

As the morning drifted on, he stayed by the windbreak, lying in the sun, eyes obscured by the darkness of his sunglasses, so we couldn't tell if he was asleep or awake. In the sea, I dared us both to swim out further and further, until our heads were bobbing in the waves.

'Edie. Don't go so far out. And look after Sophie, okay?'

His voice was as I had imagined it, as clear as the rest of the day, a memory reborn. I could sense his concern for her and wished he felt the same way about me.

'I'm okay,' she would call. She would wave back and laugh, then go under and surface again, closer. Dive, again and again. I did the same, to prove I was more daring than she was. Until he was calling both of us together. Not distinguishing.

'Hey, you two girls, come on in for a while.'

He called us over for a photograph, and we rushed to the bag to put our sunglasses on, the matching ones he had bought us. We stood with the bay as a backdrop. He tried to focus the camera, then took it away from his eye, holding it at chest height. We giggled and nudged each other as he frowned and mumbled under his breath. I would only ever half-smile, conscious of my gap. Then the photo was done. He took two cartons of juice and passed them to us.

He kissed her head, then mine, but I counted the length of the kiss, and I knew she was the special one, not me. All of the adults in my life were cold, distant. I remember feeling nothing when I thought of the words mother and father. I ran to borrow some of the love she and he shared, and, behind my sunglasses, I was weeping.

I am a twenty-nine-year-old woman, standing on an empty beach, but this runs in front of my eyes like a movie projected directly into my consciousness. It was the first summer two girls became friends, the first time we had met here at the coast, but it wasn't the last. Each summer, we grew together; eight, nine, ten. Long after Sam was no longer there. Getting taller, older. Talking, sharing. Every detail of our lives. When did it all come to an end? When did that happen? I am lost in a moment of uncertainty, as something more comes to me, something I want to push away. A jump scare; a watch-through-the-fingers moment. I watch it as an observer would. A scene crueller than I can stand, as if the film has been zoomed to an intense freeze-frame of lost innocence.

Panic in her eyes as she struggles in the sea. She is not playing this time. Do I hear myself screaming, or is it her? The picture breaks, fragments, loses focus. Then in a moment of extreme clarity I see a single image of her long brown hair, spread on the surface of the water, fanning out. Waving gently in the current like seagrass.

23

Harry

As I begin the drive back to Stowell, everything unspoken begins festering into a palpable, negative energy. One of us needs to speak, to decode this new information, but we're both mute. I look at the Somerset scenery, the fields rolling down to the coast, the wide sweep of sea and sky. The morning has come and gone; the afternoon is now wearing on. Edie stares at the hills; she hasn't looked towards the sea since we left the bay. I slow for a tractor, joining the queue of cars following it along the road.

She finally looks across at the coast, turning her shoulders to glance back the way we came. 'That day at the beach came back to me, Harry.'

I'm glad she's broken the silence first. 'Everything?'

'More or less. I remembered the photo being taken.'

'So who do you think Sophie was? A friend?'

'She was much more than that.' Now she turns to me, her eyes moist. 'And something happened to her.'

'What do you mean?'

'Something…' Her voice is so quiet I have to lean closer. 'I don't know. Something bad.'

'Edie, what did you remember?'

She is staring straight ahead now, not looking at me. 'Can a sense of guilt cause dissociation, Harry?'

'Of course, it's one of the prime factors.'

'Remember I told you that Melanie Cox refused to discuss her daughter? The one that died?'

'You think that's Sophie?'

Frustrated, she runs both hands through her hair, tugging as if trying to drag the memories out. 'Who else could she be? I remember the feeling on the beach. He was affectionate with her in the way a father would be. I felt jealous.'

'It's a reconstructed memory, Edes. It plays tricks.'

She lets a low groan of exasperation out. 'No, you don't get it. What if I've buried childhood memories because of something *I* did wrong?' She chews her already ragged cuticle. 'And the photo proves something else, too.'

I know where she's going with this. 'Your mother knew about him all along.'

'Yeah. She must have.'

'Okay, but give her the benefit of the doubt, Edes. She's been trying to protect you.'

She rounds on me angrily. 'She *knew* him, Harry. Don't you get it? Well enough to let him take me on holiday with his family.'

'The image is pretty grainy. What if we mistook—'

'It's *him*, Harry.'

She stares out the window, and I give her a moment. 'Okay. But abusers often know their victims. Your mother has clinical depression, you can't expect her to want to tell you everything. You haven't been able to face the truth of what happened either.'

She doesn't turn. The traffic chugs along at twenty as the orange lights of the tractor in front flash at us infuriatingly. I want to put my foot down and get out of this queue. There's more we need to talk about and now it has got a whole lot harder. Harder, but just as unavoidable. Her voice drags me from my thoughts.

'Harry, I want to find out what happened to Sophie. Maybe she was Samuel Cox's daughter. I'm scared though. Scared of what happened.'

'How do you mean?'

'It was the final image I remembered of Sophie in the sea. She was… face-down.'

'Drowned?'

She winces at the word and looks out of the window again at

the sea. I don't push it, and she doesn't speak for several minutes. I jump as a car speeds past the traffic line on a straight piece of road, blaring its horn. The silence deepens as Edie stares reflectively at the horizon.

'Do you know what scares me most of all?' She sighs, the subject of Sophie closed for now. She doesn't wait for a reply. 'Of becoming like my mother.'

'How do you mean?'

'Institutionalised. Mental health problems can be hereditary, can't they? I don't want to end up like her. I don't want to be labelled, categorised, imprisoned. It terrifies me.'

'No one is going to label you, Edie. You've got a condition, that's all. Lots of people who have experienced trauma or guilt suffer from repression or dissociation.'

She falls silent again. It's impossible for me to imagine her morphing into Jenny. I know institutions well, and Edie would not tolerate one. It would kill her. There is no way to imagine those green eyes, so changeable with mood and light, becoming dull, medicated; no way to imagine her skin drying out like parchment, her hair greying and thinning. She won't become her mother. I won't let it happen. But now I can understand why she kept Jenny at arm's length, even before knowing about the lies, the silence, that Jenny has infected her daughter with. The way that Edie has been manipulated by Jenny, including the most recent visit, is chilling. I wonder if our families are so different after all, despite the apparent gulf between us. Okay, my father doesn't have any skeletons in the cupboard, it's not his style. My mother is too self-obsessed to think about betrayal. But all of our psychological baggage is still there, motivating us in secret, behind the scenes.

Edie's next question is so intense and abrupt, I nearly shunt the car ahead. 'Harry, what the fuck is *wrong* with me? Tell me the truth.'

'Wrong? Nothing.'

'So why am I not frightened around the man who abducted me? Why am I even jealous of him and Sophie? Why did I feel so much guilt on that beach, as if I've done something awful?'

'Whatever you're remembering is filtered. It's not real, Edes. You were probably terrified at the time. By taking you, he would have betrayed your trust irreparably. If he was a family friend, then you're just remembering the good bits. Sifting the bad stuff out.'

'You don't get it. I've read his diary. And *I'm* the one with these feelings, not anyone else. He didn't do it, don't you see?'

'Then who did, Edes?'

'I've read between the lines. He blamed my father; he wanted to get me away from him. What if my father was the abuser, not Cox? What if Cox was trying to save me?'

'Then why does he want your forgiveness? And why did he confess?'

She shakes her head, uncertain, and lapses into silence again. We are finally pulling into the village and I swing the car into the car park of the pub. The car park is busier now, and two couples are using the outside tables. They are mine and Edie's age, laughing about something. One of the girls has her hand on her boyfriend's neck and is stroking it idly in a show of easy affection. I realise how stiff and formal Edie and I must look as we sit, staring straight ahead like we've had a blazing row.

'So what now?' I ask, turning to face her.

'What would you do?'

'Leave it. When Cox wakes up, he'll be arrested. Just stay on sick leave until then.' I hesitate, scanning her expression, watching her pick at her thumb. 'But you won't, will you?'

Her expression darkens as she stares out of the window towards the couples at the table. She knows I'm looking at her.

'No, I won't.'

'You're going to confront your mother again, aren't you?'

She nods, sucking the blood from her thumb. What did she really see at the beach? What did the memory really consist of? She's given me only as much as she wants to. Truth is a scarce commodity, but now it's my turn to share some.

I sit back in the seat, letting my head loll back, staring at the car roof.

Fuck, I mutter under my breath.

She hears, but still doesn't move. There's no more delaying this, no more time to think of a way to frame it.

'Edie, be careful if you go to see Jenny.'

She gives me a penetrating stare. 'Why?'

'There's something you should know. It's part of the reason I came here.'

'What are you on about?' Her frown deepens. I can't bear loading betrayal upon betrayal, deceit onto deceit, but I have to make sure that, if she trusts one person, it's me.

'The phone conversation with my father yesterday. It was about something that affects you. I was trying to question him about it.'

'What?' Her anxiety is growing, fused with something harder and stronger. Anger? I can feel her eyes burning into me.

Flushed, I crack the window open to let some air in. The sounds of the couples' laughter reaches us faintly. 'Edie, my father has taken a new directorship in the last few months.'

'He takes lots of directorships. He's power mad, isn't he?'

'This is different.' I twist in my seat so I'm facing her. 'My father is the new clinical director at Claydon Manor.'

24

Edie

It's been two days since I followed Harry back along the M5 towards Birmingham, my anger festering. After Harry's revelation in the car park, we had gone through the motions of analysing his father's motives for taking a directorship at Claydon Manor, even though it was blindingly obvious to me what he was doing. The post was far too much of a coincidence to be anything other than an attempt to pry into my family life. I hadn't wanted Harry at the coast in the first place, I had wanted time on my own, yet there he was. And now here's his father too, micromanaging everything, as if my being in love with his son is something that needs vetting. The thought that the need for control might be a Creighton trait has nagged at me ever since. In the end, the last thing I wanted to do is stay in Somerset and dig any further with Harry around, so I'd packed my things and, within an hour, we were both on our way home.

As soon as I reached the suburbs of the city, I'd wanted to see Jaz. Someone neutral, trustworthy. I'd arranged to meet her at work in a kind of statement of intent; call it a wilful act of rebellion if you like. So now I'm walking into the noisy cafeteria at the KG like an impostor, scanning the tables with guilty eyes. My gaze is drawn laser-like to anyone in blue scrubs, because that's what anyone who might recognise me will be wearing. Luckily, I don't see anyone to avoid. Jaz is sitting on a table half-hidden by one of the pillars, a perfect choice. I sneak across the floor of the cafeteria as if I'm playing hide-and-seek. It's not like I'm breaking some law by coming here, but I'm struggling to convince my churning stomach of that.

Then, as I walk further, a strange thing happens. The fear of discovery is lost beneath the buzz of being back at the King George again. As soon as I walked into the hospital it felt like coming home. Medicine had always been my first choice at school; I'd been so focused on getting the grades, I had almost no time for a social life. Or was that just an excuse for being so unpopular? I'd felt like Carrie in that horror film; quiet, studious, friendless, with a home life that no one else intruded on. But once I realised science came easy to me, I decided I could do without friends. When you have found a direction, something to aim for, it's easy to ride the teasing and bullying, and to ignore the comprehensive school dogma that studying is uncool. This environment is now under my skin. The hospital is where I belong, and I can't bear to be without it for much longer.

Jaz smiles as I sit down. 'How are you, hon? Is everything okay?'

'No, not really. But don't worry about it.'

'When someone says don't worry, it's usually because there's something to worry about.'

'Now's not the time, Jaz. If I started, I wouldn't stop. Honestly, it's fine. How was the date with Matt?'

She rolls her eyes dismissively, but it's a show. She liked him. 'It was okay. Nothing happened though, really.'

'You got that denial in quickly.'

'No, not on a first date. Not with a colleague, anyway. But he was different to the way he is at work. More sensitive.'

'Matt, sensitive? If you say so.' I laugh. 'Okay, so tell me what's been happening here. It feels like I've been away forever.'

'Business as usual. Morris is still a dickhead. Fiona is still a lazy cow. And yes, Matt does still need mothering. But we miss you, Edie.'

'Has Morris talked about me?'

She tilts her head. That's her sympathy look. 'Ah. Don't take this the wrong way, but for him it's like you never existed. But he is completely anal, as you know. He wouldn't talk about things like that anyway; he'd keep whatever he thought to himself.'

'Never existed? Really?' I slump back in my chair, and gaze up at the high, domed ceiling. I close my eyes. 'They want me out for good, I can feel it.'

'No. They can't do that.'

'Morris is regretting taking me on.'

She sighs, hesitating. She knows how Morris and I clash, and she has listened to my complaints about what I call the Morris–Wilson tag team for months. 'That's not true.'

'Jaz, that pause was far too long.' She looks embarrassed, so I don't press her. 'So what about our guy then?'

She whistles, low and long, her eyes gleaming. 'Cox? You wouldn't believe it, Edie; he is still improving. They're weaning him off the inotropes, his urine output is half-decent. I mean, his liver is still struggling, but it's functioning.'

'Will they wake him up?'

'You know what Morris is like, he keeps his cards close to his chest. Cox's wounds have healed, we've stopped the antibiotics. He's still marked and scarred, of course.' She shrugs. 'Put it this way: if he keeps improving, it'll be a matter of days until we have the pleasure of his company.'

Since Harry and I got back from the coast the day before yesterday, I've been torn by indecision. Claydon Manor has haunted me to the point where I haven't been able to think rationally about what to do. Harry explained that after letting slip about the directorship, his father had backtracked quickly. The directorship was offered, his father claimed, so he took it. He didn't actively seek it. But that's nonsense; these positions aren't just offered. He had accused Harry of being paranoid, hinted that I was turning him against his own father. Harry is stuck in the middle like me. He won't admit openly to being too browbeaten to accuse his father of meddling, but sometimes – just occasionally – he will let the façade slip, and I can see the anger. A hint of what goes on behind his poker face.

So now I'm paralysed by doubt. Caught between wanting to see my mother and my desperation to avoid James Creighton. The thought of getting past Sue Willard, the nurse in charge at Claydon

Manor, doesn't fill me with joy either. If one certainty has come out of this revelation, it's that Harry's father and I are never going to be reconciled, which makes things worse. At least in Jaz I have someone to talk to with no connection to Harry or his obnoxious family.

'Jaz, I've got something to tell you. You know Samuel Cox abducted me when I was eight? That he was supposed to have abused me?' She flinches at the word *abused*. 'I have to say it, Jaz. It happened, so I'm told.'

She nods. 'I guess. It just upsets me on your behalf. Yes, I know what was in the papers, Edie.'

'Well, since being put on sick leave, I've visited the village where he took me.'

'Are you serious? Why?'

'I don't have a choice. I can't just sit at home, can I?' I hesitate, picking my next words carefully. It's hard to have kept things from your best friend, and I don't know how she will take it. 'Jaz, I haven't told you everything.'

'Okaayy.' Her voice drips with uncertainty, her eyes full of concern.

'Before I was put on sick leave, I went to see Samuel Cox's wife Melanie. She gave me his diary; inside was a photo of me and another girl called Sophie on a beach. I was going to tell you all this at the pub.'

'Oh, Edie. How deep into this have you got?'

'Deep enough to know that Samuel Cox knew me, and believed my father Michael was the abuser.' I suck in a deep breath. There's no going back after admitting this. 'And I think he's telling the truth. I saw the cottage he took me to, and I felt no fear of the place at all. We found the beach in the photo too. All I remembered was affection for him. Love, almost. Not fear though.'

'Edie…'

'No, listen. I can't prove this because I don't remember the abuse, but, when he implies it was my father who did it, I believe him.'

The doubt in her eyes unnerves me. 'Edie. Predators make excuses all the time. It's *never* their fault, is it?'

'Samuel Cox *knew* me, Jaz. Before he took me.'

'Oh, hon. No wonder your nerves are so frayed.'

I lapse into silence. Though Jaz and I share everything, I can't tell her about that intense, hyper-real image of Sophie's dark hair, waving back and forth in the swaying current of deep water. I want to push it away, as if something unforgivable has happened. In the shock after the visit to the beach I was almost too honest with Harry, but I've tried not to think about it since. I'm being set adrift, while still trying to hold on to my old life, the one where things were reassuringly predictable. I never realised how much I liked predictability. Trying to keep the old me in sight is like clinging to a waft of smoke as it blows away in the breeze.

'I don't know what to think any more, Jaz. What if he was wrongly convicted?'

'Edie, stop looking for things that aren't there. I'm worried about you.' Maybe Jaz thinks her pity is helping but all it does is confirm how disorientated I feel. Her gaze is designed to tell me she understands. But she doesn't, not really. She pushes a stray lock back from her brow, pulls her ponytail tighter. 'He knew you, so what? Why would that stop him being an abuser?'

'I don't know, but it's just how I feel. All I've got to go on are the memories that are coming back to me. About me *and* Sophie. About him too. Some of them are clearer than others.'

'Fine, let's say an innocent man confessed for some reason. *Why?*'

'I don't know.' The cafeteria is getting busier, the noise and clatter is too loud, too grating. 'I want to find out more about Sophie. I think she was Cox's daughter. His wife says she's dead, and I need to find out.'

'How?'

'My mother.' There's the shadow of Claydon Manor again. There is the imposing heaviness of those walls. The smell. The strained atmosphere of politeness, underscored with the threat of control. The doors, the locks. 'I need to ask her what she knows. But something else has happened. I don't trust Harry's family.'

'What do you mean?'

'It's Harry's father. He's…' I realise I haven't told Jaz yet about my mother being a voluntary inpatient at Claydon Manor. Now is not the time. 'Let's just say James Creighton is a meddling creep.'

Her brown eyes widen. 'Harry's father's first name is James?'

'Yeah, why?'

'Older, greying guy? Looks a bit like a playboy who's past his sell-by date?'

'That's one way of putting it.'

She watches me carefully, gauging my reaction. 'It's an unusual surname, and I knew Harry's father was a psychiatrist. But I just didn't put two and two together. I didn't think—'

'Think what?' I interrupt. 'Jaz, for God's sake, tell me.'

'There was a conference here, at the postgraduate centre. James Creighton was one of the speakers. He was in the ICU chatting to Morris like they're old friends.'

I try to form a reply, but my mouth isn't obeying my brain. I manage a single word. 'What?'

At that moment, my phone buzzes on the table. Jaz and I both look down at the same time. As we register the name on the screen, I stare at her, my grip on reality slipping. It can't be. I let it buzz, vibrating against the hard surface.

'Speak of the bloody devil,' Jaz hisses. 'Are you going to answer it?'

I look down again; it has rung four times already; it will cut off in the next two rings unless I answer. But the name flashing out of the screen has turned me to stone.

James Creighton.

Jaz nods at the phone urgently. *Go on*, she mouths.

As the phone is about to cut to voicemail, my finger finds the screen and swipes across to accept the call. As though I'm gripping a stick of lit dynamite, I hold the phone to my ear, and answer it in a hoarse whisper.

'Hello?'

'Hello, Edie.' His voice is its usual deep, measured drawl. 'It's time we had a chat, don't you think?'

25

Harry

The Emergency Department is hectic as usual. I make my way through the crowds and find the cubicle where Georgia, an eighteen-year-old girl with anorexia, is curled up on her trolley in a foetal position. She is my third emergency psychiatric referral of the day. I glance at her notes, then at the figure under the blankets. Her weight of 39 kilograms is obvious in the only part of her I can see above the covers; her face is narrow, her pale eyes wide and hollow, watching me as I come in. How did it get to this? Why was her condition not picked up months earlier, before this crisis happened? I explain as gently as I can that she will need to be treated as an inpatient until we can get her calorie intake stabilised, but the fear is already in her eyes at the thought of giving up control of what she puts in her body.

I'm holding the emergency bleep until eight this evening and the handover can't come soon enough. Edie's panicked phone call at lunchtime has been running through my head, and every single permutation I can think of is bad. My father wanted to meet her, alone. He will come to the house when I was out, he told her. I don't fear for her physically – it's not as if my father is going to hurt her – but I'm pissed off I can't second-guess his motives. I've never heard Edie so flustered. *What does he want? What's it about?* She was fixating on rhetorical questions, talking incessantly, convinced he was going to find a way to get her sacked. I tried telling her he didn't have that kind of power, but I couldn't hide the doubt in my voice. She wouldn't hear of me talking to my father beforehand to find out what it was about, because he had specifically said he wanted the conversation to be private. She'd rung off, saying she wanted time to collect her thoughts, which for Edie means brooding, worrying, and overthinking.

So now, I'm counting the minutes until my colleague Amad takes the emergency bleep from me, so I can get home. But Georgia's case is dragging on, and I want some closure before I go. I spend nearly an hour on the phone trying to make referrals, doing my best to get her into an eating disorders centre, but the nearest one with a bed is in Manchester. Her parents look horrified at this; neither of them can afford to travel that far to visit her and she'd be more isolated than ever. Perhaps I'm tired, but it bugs me that she might just be sent home in a few days and end up joining a long queue for a few CBT sessions. Stabilised, then sent home to get sick again. Finally, I admit defeat, and spend the next twenty minutes explaining to her I'll get something put in place over the next few days.

It's nearly nine before I finally hand the bleep over to Amad and slalom my way back through the Emergency Department. Swearing under my breath, I realise I've left my phone in my office, and walk across the car park to get it, enjoying the cool evening air.

As I bleep myself onto the administrative floor, I'm immediately wary. The corridor is empty and silent, as I'd expect it to be at nine in the evening, but at the far end yellow light is escaping from beneath one of the office doors. No one ever stays in this part of the building as late as this; anyone who is on shift overnight always works from the offices attached to the secure unit, which is staffed permanently. By seven, once the cleaners have clicked all the lights off, this floor usually remains undisturbed until eight the following morning, when the administrative staff begin drifting in. I let myself into my office, picking up my phone from the desk, checking it for messages. Nothing. Without turning the main lights on, I move along the corridor towards the far office. Maybe a cleaner left the light switched on, I try to convince myself. The old building is eerie enough in the daytime, but now, in the gloom, it is sending a shiver up even my sceptical spine.

I realise the light is coming from Amy Wilson's office, a fan of warm yellow spreading out from the gap beneath the door, shining on the wooden floor of the corridor. Despite the light, the whole floor still has that unnerving feeling of being empty. Without even thinking of knocking, I grab the handle.

Then, in the single movement it takes to turn the handle and push, several things happen at once. I'm aware of noises coming from beyond the door. The unmistakable low noises of quiet, furtive sex.

As the handle turns, there is a hurried shout from inside. Male, loud and shocked.

A flustered exclamation, barely intelligible.

Wait.

There is a muffled female voice, which yells something incoherent. But it's too late and the door swings inwards. Then it's open, and there they both are.

The first thought that occurs to me is: why the fuck didn't they lock it?

In the corner, Amy Wilson is hurriedly pulling her skirt down, her blouse untucked. She smooths her hair as she tries to cross the floor with some decorum, striding from the couch towards the door.

Facing away from us, as if he is trying to stare through the closed curtains and out into the night, is Richard Morris, pushing his shirt back into his half-mast trousers. There is the metallic jingle of a belt buckle as he fumbles with the clasp.

When he has it secure, he turns and looks at me, red-faced. Equally flushed, I mutter a garbled apology and pull the door closed again, the sight of Wilson and Morris in panicked *coitus interruptus* burned into my mind. The door was open for less than five seconds, but it's left me with an image I can never unsee. I've met Amy Wilson's husband several times at department functions. He's an academic; quiet and studious, and in his small stature, intense stare and quick movements a male version of Amy herself. Morris's family are just abstract archetypes to me, although Edie has said how stiff and formal they look from the photos in his office, just like those sepia Victorian parlour images where the husband's hand rests possessively on his wife's crinoline-clad shoulder. I wonder how many formalities there would be if either Daniel Wilson or Tina Morris could see their flustered spouses now. So much for doctors being trustworthy.

Resisting the urge to break into an impulsive run, I walk as fast as I can away from the office, desperate to get out of there. I'm halfway along the corridor, aiming for the security-controlled door to the stairs, when Wilson's office door opens again, and I hear the quick tick-tick-tick of her heels as she runs along the corridor after me.

'Harry?' she calls. 'Wait.' I pause and turn. She has regained her composure, although it would be impossible to be *less* composed than she was a moment ago. She has even put her suit jacket back on. 'Harry. That was…' She sighs, briefly lost for words. 'Inappropriate. I'm not sure what I can say to you.'

'It's none of my business, Amy,' I tell her.

'No.' She pauses again. 'But you won't say anything, will you?'

I fight a losing battle to maintain eye contact. She is a colleague, and although I don't know Morris professionally I know how closely he works with Edie, so I'm conflicted by this conversation on so many levels. All I can do is repeat myself. 'Honestly, it's none of my business.'

She nods, still flushed. I allow myself a half-smile, something between conciliatory and embarrassed, then I turn again and leave as quickly as dignity will let me.

The night air feels even better now, even cooler on my face, which is still burning with embarrassment; for both them *and* me. The absurdity of the scene imprinted on my brain hits me, and as the shock ebbs away I smile again, this time with a wild, half-manic grin. And to think I'd always considered Amy Wilson boring. Then I'm laughing incredulously, in a quick release of shock and disbelief.

I head towards the car, now in even more of a rush to get home. I'm no gossip, but there's no way I'm going to be able to keep this secret from Edie; it's far too juicy. With everything that's gone on, now more than ever she needs some salacious scandal to cheer her up.

26
Edie

Harry had made me swear not to tell Jaz, and I'd agreed reluctantly. Picturing what he'd seen between Wilson and Morris had made me feel simultaneously amused, nauseous and livid. Their little double act with the woman from HR was now so transparent it was insulting. How dare they sit there and pass judgement on my fitness to work, when they're fucking each other behind everyone's backs?

Their arrogance, their smugness, which was so grating when they put me on sick leave, has now become outright hypocrisy. Although Harry and I laughed and made puerile jokes at their expense, underneath I was boiling with anger, as our conversation alternated between our two-faced colleagues and our messed-up parents. We hadn't managed to come to any agreement on what his father wanted, and I hadn't felt able to tell him what my plans for today were either. I knew he'd try to dissuade me.

I'd waited until Harry left for work and then mentally prepared myself. The drive to Claydon Manor has taken me an hour, which has been valuable thinking time. As the sign for the village of Nether Claydon approaches, I wonder what they think of having a psychiatric unit on their doorstep; the village looks like the kind of place where NIMBYs abound. Yet more hypocrisy; how many sociopathic businessmen, narcissistic executives and barely coping housewives or househusbands are living in denial behind these rose-framed doors and large, immaculate frontages? I turn into the grounds of Claydon Manor, the tyres crunching on the gravel drive, which winds through the gardens towards the ornate, Gothic main entrance. I scan the car park for James Creighton's Tesla. It's not there. Consciously slowing my breathing, adopting my professional air, I report to reception.

As ever, Sue Willard is doing an uncanny impersonation of Nurse Ratched in that old Jack Nicholson film. Perhaps it's the pinched lips, the cold, grey stare, or the air of the strict head girl that makes her such a dead ringer. Even though the uniform in these places is usually casual – in Claydon's case a green polo shirt and trousers – Willard still carries it off with an aura of frigid, air-conditioned detachment.

'I wish you'd called first, Edie. This is a bit irregular.' She uses the subsequent silence effectively, but I hold my nerve. The entire journey here has been a battle of insecurity versus willpower, and now I'm not in the mood to follow her script. Eventually, with a quick glance at the bunch of flowers I'm holding, she continues in her passive-aggressive drawl. 'Of course, you're more than welcome to see her though.'

'Thank you. And yes, I'm sorry I came at short notice. Something cropped up earlier today, and I need to speak to my mother about it.'

She gives me an angular, lupine smile. 'Is it something I can help you with?'

As she's manager of the unit, I'm suspicious of Willard by default. She will know who the new clinical director is by now and will probably have already met him. My prospective father-in-law. My answer is quick and definite. 'No, I'd rather talk to her myself.'

She smiles again, with upbeat insincerity. 'Okay, perhaps for a short while then. Follow me.'

Willard leads me along the corridor to my mother's room. Inside, she is sitting in an easy chair, staring out of the window towards the distant hills. In this place she looks more shrunken, more withdrawn, than she ever did at home. Willard waits by the door, watching us, until the silence drags on long enough for her to get the hint. The door clicks quietly shut and my mother and I are alone. I sit opposite, following her gaze out towards the hills where shadows of the fast-moving clouds are scudding along the slopes and valleys. I dip my head, finding her eyes, fixing her gaze.

'Hello, Mum. These are for you.' She stares listlessly at the flowers, her eyes flat. I stand up, still playing the charade of the dutiful, visiting daughter. 'I'll put them in something, shall I?' I wander around the room, checking cupboards for a vase. 'How have you been?' I call brightly over my shoulder. There's no answer, and my half-hearted search ends with me laying the flowers on her bed as if someone had died there.

Finally, when I sit back down again, she speaks. Her eyes have not moved from the scenery outside. 'Edie, this has upset me.'

'Please don't be like that,' I say, leaning forward. She sighs as if about to reply but then lapses back into silence, still avoiding my gaze. I try again. 'Mum, why don't you ever look at me? Listen, we need to talk.'

She finally turns. 'Talk? About what?'

'You know what about, Mum. You can't hide in here from what's happened.'

'I said you should leave it.'

'I can't. Not any more.' I think of James Creighton's unexpected call yesterday. His measured voice. *I'll come to your house. So make sure my son is out.* Okay, Professor Creighton, we'll talk, but I need to know what you're up to first. I rest my hand on my mother's stick-thin arm. 'Mum, has a new doctor been to see you recently? An older man, distinguished looking?'

She nods, a shadow clouding her face, mirroring the landscape. 'He says he wants to help us.'

I try to identify the sensation in the centre of my chest. Is it fear? Rage? Both? 'Have you said anything to him? About us? About me?'

'I don't think so. I get so confused.'

'Mum, why won't you face what's going on? I have to.'

'Oh, I know what's happening.' A rare flash of life surfaces in her eyes before sinking into the depths again. 'Our lives are falling apart.'

'Not if I can help it. Look, he doesn't have our best interests at heart. That's why I need to know whether you've said anything to him?'

'No. I don't trust him.' She eyes me suspiciously.

'Good. Neither do I.' I don't push the fact she hasn't spoken to me either. 'You need to know something about him. He's Harry's father. He wants to split Harry and me up. I don't know why he hates me so much.' I stroke her hand. It is unbearably frail. On my free hand, the fingernail digs into the quick of my thumb again, as if it wants to rip it off. That old habit.

She glances down at the sudden movement. 'You haven't done that for years.'

I force myself to stop. 'Look, I've found some things out since we last met.'

'I don't want to know any more.' Her attention returns to the landscape, avoiding my gaze. 'Edie, I just wanted the best for you.'

'Why won't you look at me? What are you hiding?' It's too late to spare her feelings now. We've been sparing each other for too long, and there's too much at stake. 'Samuel Cox was a friend of our family, wasn't he?'

'No, Samuel Cox ruined everything.' Beneath my mother's frown, a quiet, unseen battle is raging. It has been going on for years, ever since she became a single mother. She has tried to manage for both of us, tried to balance how she feels against what she thinks I can bear to know. She is constantly finding that compromise. We should have talked long ago, before the cracks widened like glacial fissures. The distance between us echoes in the vitriol of her next words. She fixes me with a glittering, malicious stare. 'You've become the proper little detective, haven't you? Where do you find the time?'

I ignore the petulance. 'I'm going to tell you what I know, and you need to listen. We're the only ones who can help each other.'

As I talk, she stares silently at the landscape, the window reflecting her face, as the gathering clouds meet and build over the hills. I tell her about the bay, about finding the cottage. I remind her about Melanie Cox, the journal. I don't hold anything back, because I want her to remember that the past, the one that she and I hold somewhere inside of us, is for us alone to resolve, and no one else. It is not for James Creighton to use like a weapon to prove we're damaged, or to demonstrate that I'm not good enough for his son, his family, or that I'm not stable enough to be a doctor. Whatever he has against me, I can't let him win. Men like him *always* win.

The rain begins to fall, and my mother sits so still it's as if she herself is part of a faded snapshot, some moment long past. As rivulets pour down the windowpane, the hills and fields beyond the walls of Claydon Manor become greyer, mistier. Finally, I tell her the truth; that I think Samuel Cox is innocent. That he didn't do all those things he confessed to. No one else believes me; I wonder if she will? When I finish speaking, I have to lean close to hear her voice.

'Edie, I'm so sorry.' She is looking beyond me, through me and into the past, as though she is imagining me as an eight-year-old girl again. But she will not meet my gaze. 'I'm sorry for everything.'

'Mum, look at me. I'm here. What happened to us?'

'Let's just go away again. You and me.' She leans close and kisses me on the cheek, holding me near to her. Near to her thin hair, a side effect of the medication, near the papery, cool skin of her fingers. I hold her too. I'm sorry as well, Mum. Sorry for all the pain and the guilt we've suffered. She holds my face gently near hers, her eyes inches from mine. I can smell the coffee on her, the sickly sweetness of her breath. 'Let's run away.'

I gently ease myself from her grasp. 'No, we can't run this time. It's too late. You need to tell me about Samuel Cox.'

'Samuel Cox took you. He hurt you. It was all in the papers.'

'No, Samuel Cox was innocent, wasn't he? He blames Dad for the abuse.' She turns away, lips drawn together. 'Mum, what was going on at home to make him take me away? What did my father do to me?'

'Stop it, please.'

'What happened at the coast? What happened to Sophie?'

'Stop it.' More insistent, sharper. 'If you're not careful, you'll be in here with me.'

In there with her? The thought stops me dead. I think of James Creighton and my stomach flips. It would be an extreme way to rid yourself of an unwanted daughter-in-law, but *what if*? What if he's capable of putting us both here? I push the thought away. This isn't the Victorian era; I don't care how powerful he is, or how many connections he has, he can't just lock people up on a whim.

'Mum, why was Samuel Cox suspicious of Dad? I read it in his diary, it's all there. He hated Dad for something, didn't he? Why? What happened before I was taken?'

As my mother stares at me, time freezes. It is like looking at a stranger. She is becoming agitated, her voice louder. 'My husband is dead. Why can't you just let him rest in peace?'

'I'm not the only one who's going to be asking you these questions. Creighton will too. You'd better get used to that.'

Her voice is becoming shrill; she turns away. 'Michael was violent. He was a difficult man, but you would always anger him. *Provoke* him.'

'Provoke him to do what? Why are you still making excuses for him?'

'Haven't you done enough?' she screams, turning back, her eyes blazing through the medication. 'Aren't enough lives ruined?'

I sit back as the force of her rage disperses, leaving her breathing hard. My chest is thumping with the sudden outburst. In the silence, the door clicks open, and a man comes into the room without knocking. I tense even further, until I see the man is in his late twenties, dressed casually in shirt and trousers with a man bun and scrubby beard. Not Creighton, thank God. Around his neck an identification card hangs from a green lanyard. *Kieran McMillan – Nurse.*

'Everything okay, guys?' Kieran asks. 'I heard raised voices.' My mother has lapsed into a wary silence.

'Yes, we're fine.' I draw my hand across my forehead and look across at her lined face, her limp hair falling across her brow. Whatever had burned in her eyes is now gone, and she looks exhausted. A pang of guilt hits me at pushing her like this, but I had to. Others will push her too, harder. And they will have no conscience. They don't love her like I do.

'Time for lunch, Mrs Carter,' Kieran tells her, looking at me. 'Sorry, you'll have to go, I'm afraid.'

I lean down to give my mother a kiss on the cheek. She lets me, as if her outburst never happened. She still couldn't be honest with me, even now, but I know for sure that I was right. It was in her eyes. Samuel Cox may have taken me, but he didn't do anything to me. He's innocent of the abuse they locked him up for. He loved me, I'm certain of it.

Of course, the abuse happened, the reports showed that, so they pinned it on Cox and he didn't deny it. Why, though? Why serve nearly twenty years for a crime you didn't commit? In the diaries, he points the finger, and it's obvious who he blames. What would the police have made of those insinuations if they had seen them at the time? A horrible thought occurs to me; surely Melanie Cox didn't keep those diaries secret as a way of punishing her husband?

But if Cox was right, it was my father, who I can't even remember, who inflicted the emotional damage on me that came out in the reports.

As my lips brush against my mother's skin, I glance at Kieran, hovering near the door. My voice is no more than a whisper, but I know she can hear it.

'Mum, let me take you home.'

She shakes her head. *No.* 'I'm staying.'

'When he comes, don't tell him anything.'

Her nod is brief, almost indiscernible, but it's enough.

27

Harry

As I wait on the landing in the dark, listening for the doorbell, I can't believe what Edie has talked me into. A supposedly private meeting with my father, and she's convinced me to listen in. I can't work out why it should bother me so much; it's in my interests to know what my father wants to say to her. My anxious, guilt-ridden upbringing has taught me a whole range of values and patterns of behaviour that are complete bollocks when you analyse them. Eavesdropping is devious. Boys don't cry. Stiff upper lip. Death before dishonour. I have schoolfriends now working in the City who think nothing of asset-stripping a company or manipulating stocks, but would die of shame if they let the team down at rugby. What crap.

Yesterday, Edie returned home in the middle of a filthy evening, soaked from the storm which had been lashing the West Midlands for hours, and had flatly refused to say where she'd been. I let it go, just as I didn't mention the fact she'd obviously been crying. When she shouted that her time was her own, and she could do what the fuck she liked with it, instead of fighting back like I wanted to, I placated her. *Of course. You do this at your own pace, Edes.* I made her a drink and we talked about my father and why he might want to see her. It took us less than half a glass before we were arguing, skirting around what we now understood to be the truth; my father doesn't like her. *Big deal*, I'd said. There are lots of in-laws for whom their son- or daughter-in-law will never be good enough. She had always claimed it was a class thing, that just because my family are privileged they want me to marry someone of my own social status.

148

But as I was denying it, I knew every word she was saying was true. *Okay, my family are fucking snobs*, I finally yelled. *Happy now?*

Edie has a way of teasing some twisted logic out of a situation, and of turning the irrational into the only reasonable course of action, and that's why I'm now crouching up here in the dark like a burglar. It will be interesting to hear the fireworks if nothing else; my father might think he has the measure of Edie Carter, but he's in for a shock. I know her better than him, and mine is a knowledge born out of love. His is born of prejudice. I can look behind those green eyes, and unravel the thoughts and follow the spiderwebs of synapses that make her who she is. I know why she is driven; I know why she is ambitious, and I also know that, in her, my father has butted up against another control freak. Perhaps I'm getting her to fight my battles, say what I could never say to him, but even a coward can enjoy watching a good fight once in a while.

When the bell rings and Edie shows him into the kitchen, I creep downstairs and put my ear against the door. Their voices carry clearly, hers quiet and resolute, his clipped and precise. I'm standing where Edie would have been when she heard me on the phone before she left for the coast. They exchange a curt greeting and a stool grates against the tiles as someone sits on it, presumably him. Then silence. I let the breath I've been holding out in a controlled hiss. My father speaks first.

'I expect you're wondering why I wanted to see you?'

'It had crossed my mind, James, yes.'

There is an icy pause from him at her use of his first name. He always insisted she should call him James, in that polite way he has, yet he never seemed to like her doing it. That's where his sense of etiquette rubs up against his hypocrisy.

'But you know why really, don't you?'

'No. Enlighten me.'

'Well, Edie. It's quite simple really. A few days ago, I had a conference at the King George. I took the opportunity to—'

'To talk to Richard Morris about me?' I imagine his look of indignation; no one interrupts my father.

When his voice rumbles through the gap again, it's less assured. 'Yes, how did you know?'

'I still know people at the hospital. I'm not completely cut off, you know.'

'Well, I suppose it's no secret. It was never meant to be.'

The power balance is delicately poised. It's amazing what you can tell from tone of voice alone. 'And you discussed Samuel Cox?' Edie asks.

'We discussed lots of things.'

'And you talked about what he supposedly did to me?'

A pause, a microsecond. 'As I said, we discussed lots of things.'

'I bet you did.' There is a steely edge to her voice, a mixture of indignation and bitterness coming from a sense of injustice. For Edie, it's always men like my father who have the power to influence the world, to move the pieces on the chessboard, and she hates them for it. 'Because that's what you do, James. You decide on others' futures, make decisions about people like me. It's power, isn't it? You're desperate to know all about my past.'

'Am I really?'

'Your new clinical directorship at Claydon Manor suggests so.'

'Ah, so my sensitive son has been unable to keep his powder dry. Well, I've had many senior positions, young lady,' he replies coolly. 'This is just one of them.'

His condescending tone will be winding her up no end, but she pushes on. 'And is it the role of the director to medicate patients? To interrogate them?'

The stool slides backwards, scraping on the tiles again, and my body tenses. He must have stood up; his voice is low, dangerously low. 'That's a very serious accusation, Doctor Carter. You need to think carefully about what you say.'

'Well, I'm sorry if I'm not quite as measured as the great Professor,' she spits. 'Not quite as… fucking bloodless.'

In the pause that follows, I picture my father smoothing his hair back like the pantomime villain, folding his arms in front of him, resting the elbows of his Anderson & Sheppard suit on the wooden top of the breakfast bar. 'Don't lose your temper. You don't see me losing mine, do you?'

No, you will rarely see him losing his temper, not these days. But be careful, Edie, because it's in there. Take it from me, he is deliberately provoking you now.

'So why did you want to talk?' After her outburst she now sounds sullen. 'You already seem to know everything about me.'

'I'll come straight to the point, shall I?'

'I wish you would.'

'All right. I want you away from my son. For good.'

And there it is. Proof of everything she has ever said to me. Proof of everything I've denied for the past two years. For a moment I know the true meaning of red mist, as my reasoning is replaced by an overpowering urge to stride into the kitchen and knock the inevitable smug expression from his face. My fists bunch, white-knuckled. Then sanity kicks back in. My nerve fails, as it always does. Instead I wait, my hearing so acute the ticking of the clock near the front door sounds like a drumbeat. My father's words are measured and precise.

'And if you end the relationship, I will go no further in my...' He pauses, and even through the heavy wooden door I can feel the atmosphere thicken. I picture them holding each other's gaze, neither wanting to blink first.

'In your what, James?' She is barely audible.

'In my investigation. My *probe* into your mental health. Into your suitability, as it were. Both as a doctor and a partner for my son. I don't have to elaborate, do I?' She doesn't reply, and there is another loaded pause. 'So, do you agree?'

'No. Of course not. Why would I agree to that?'

'Because you know what I can do. I can ruin your life. Pull it down brick by brick. Dismantle everything you've built. You surely understand that, at least?'

Silence. Why isn't she screaming at him, bawling him out? Where are you, Edie, where has your fight gone? Finally, she replies. She sounds as if she's being choked. 'That would be unethical. You can't use your position like that.'

'Try me. This is the only means I have to get you two apart. I've spoken to your consultant. The man who signs your papers, ticks your boxes, makes your decisions. I can make sure you never get your job back. Once I'm done with you, the stigma will follow you for the rest of whatever pathetic career you can build from the wreckage. I know what you want, Doctor Carter. I know what you've fought so hard to get.' He is now pure business, no emotion. Running the show. 'And I know what frightens you most, too.'

Nothing is said while the moment holds. I soften my breathing. Edie's response is barely more than a whisper. 'I'm a good doctor. I've worked hard to get where I am.'

'So have I,' he replies. 'I have spent years building a reputation – my own and my son's – which I will not see jeopardised. You and my son will never see each other again. You will make an excuse to leave him; I don't care what it is.' He becomes emphatic; I picture him leaning forward, jaw square. 'I want you out of my son's life. And then I'll get out of yours. Do you agree?'

Everything I ever felt about my father now ignites in a fierce, blazing fire of loathing deep in my core. My mother is weak, but I can forgive her for that. Maybe it's her I've inherited this yellow streak from where he's concerned. She has managed to stay married to this arsehole of a man all these years by finding her own form of coping. Like me, she would rather push it away than stand up to him. My anger and bitterness spill out in other ways; she self-medicates for hers. I've seen the Temazepam on her bedside table when she forgot to hide it. Noticed the clock-watching until five each evening and her first drink. Witnessed her dreamy, robotic expression. She has kept herself sedated, exactly like Edie's mother. But for families like mine, it's a little secret to be hidden. Just a cure for a touch of everyday misery.

But my father is a different breed. Calculating, measured. He finds weakness and preys on it.

He is now loud, persuasive. The voice of the natural deal-closer. The politician. 'I said do you agree, Edie?'

I wait for her reply. Where is the anger, the outrage? Where is the frustration at being manipulated? What can he have on her to pull this kind of stunt? No, she will fight, she will tell him where to go. She won't sacrifice what we have together for her career. She won't let him get one over on her.

Her voice is quiet, but in her own way she is just as firm as him. Just as decisive.

'Yes,' she states simply. 'I agree.'

28

Edie

'Edie, what have you just done?' Before I can slide the safety latch across on the front door after Creighton leaves, Harry is thundering back down the stairs. He stands close to me, breathing hard. 'I mean, seriously? What the actual fuck?'

Without replying, I slip past him, ignoring his wide-eyed, confused stare, and head to the kitchen. His shadow follows me as I stand with my back to him and pour the biggest glass of wine in the world. I'm still shaking as I guide the lip of the bottle to the glass.

'Do you want one?' I ask.

'What? No, I want an answer.'

The wine catches the light as I pour. Harry has always thought my preference for Pinot Grigio blush was a tad – how can one put it – *common*. I once tried to take some to a Creighton family gathering, and when we got there I discovered he'd swapped it for a bottle of Malbec. I take a big slug of my cheap pink wine; as far as I'm concerned, the whole Creighton family and their snobbery can do one right now.

'Edie? What are you playing at?'

I keep my eyes on the wall; not because I don't want to look at him, but because I don't want to answer until I've calmed down. After a few seconds of loaded silence I turn. Surprisingly, my voice is steady. 'You should ask your father what he's doing, Harry, not me. You should ask him why he wants me out of your life so badly. Why he's been asking Morris and Wilson about me.'

He is shaking his head, his eyes wounded. 'Because he's an interfering bastard. But how could you just agree to it? He hasn't got anything on you. How could you finish us like that?'

Why can't he see what I can see? Why does he have to be so literal? 'I haven't *finished* us, Harry. I would never do that.'

He tugs his fingers through his wavy, dark hair, clutching a fistful of it with a groan of frustration, wheeling away. 'Edie. What kind of games are you playing? These are my fucking emotions we're talking about.'

'They're mine too.' I take my wine across to the breakfast bar and sit back on the same stool I sat on to talk to Creighton. Harry sits opposite, still supporting his head with bunched fists.

'I don't get why you're doing this,' he groans. 'I don't understand.'

'Yes, you do, Harry. I think what's bothering you is you knew all along it was going to come to this somehow. He will never accept me – he'll go to any lengths to get me away from you.'

He puffs his cheeks out and rubs his eyes with the ball of his hand. Now the adrenaline has ebbed out of my system, all that's left is a deep, enduring affection for the man opposite. How exactly does it feel when a boy sees a father in his true light? Is it like the bereavement I felt when my mother drifted away from me into her dark places? Just like me, he has done his best to keep believing in his parents. You do, don't you? That's the problem. No matter how much the evidence tells you they are weak and flawed, or liars and bullies, you still want to believe in them. I take his hand across the breakfast bar, but he pulls it away petulantly.

'No, Edie. You just agreed to never see me again, don't get all affectionate.'

I bristle at the snub; how does he know so little of me? 'Sorry to ruin my good girl image, Harry, but I am capable of lying too, you know.' I lean forward. 'Come on. You still don't get your father's game, do you? It's a power play, nothing more. So we let him think he's won.'

'Maybe you should explain it to me like I'm a three-year-old? Seeing how this doesn't seem to bother you.'

'Listen, I have less than three months to go before my final exams. He is tight with Morris, and more importantly with Wilson. His influence is definitely enough to put my progression in doubt if I don't play along. But it doesn't mean I actually have to make that choice.'

'For fuck's sake. There are other jobs, aren't there?'

'Of course not. Your father's not stupid. He knows my background, how hard I've worked to get this far. Wilson hates me, I've been resistant all the way through this. You must know the GMC fitness to practise rules? It only takes two consultant psychiatrists to declare a doctor unfit. Your father is just trading one thing for another. It's the way people like him work.'

'Okay, our careers are important. But I love you, Edie – you don't seem to understand how much. Why do you care so much if he researches you and your mother anyway?'

'Oh God, Harry. Really?' How can he be so blind? Having heard what his father said, he still believes there are boundaries James Creighton won't cross to get his own way. 'I saw a side of him this evening that scares the hell out of me. You were only listening; I *saw* in his eyes what he was prepared to do.'

'Like what, exactly?'

'Question my competence, imply I'm unstable. Get me fired.' I pause, finally framing the words I can barely whisper to myself. 'Section me.'

'Section you? Oh, come on. He doesn't have that much power, Edes.'

I roll my eyes. Why does privilege never recognise itself? 'Harry, if he, Morris and Wilson all decide to pull their weight, I'm done. I don't want my fucking sanity questioned either, okay? Your father, with his old-school-tie influence, can make all of that happen.'

A groan escapes him. 'He's a prick. But he wouldn't go that far.'

'Now who's the one in denial? I saw my mother yesterday. *That's* where I went, okay? She's medicated, Harry. Heavily medicated and scared. He's been pressing her for information on me. He is looking for reasons to prove me unfit.'

He looks down at his hands. His defence of his father was brief and half-hearted. It says it all; he knows him better than anyone. He sighs. 'Okay. Let's say he is capable of doing all those things. Where does that leave us then? We need each other, Edie.'

'We play his game. We make a show of splitting up, but stay together.'

'For how long?'

'Until I'm qualified. Then we take off somewhere else, and can do whatever we want.'

'Gaslight my own father?' He motions to the bottle on the worktop, and I pour him some more, standing over him as I put the glass by his hand. He looks at it, then swallows half. 'Your choice of wine is still shit, by the way.'

'Thanks.' I smile, but he is stony-faced. 'There's something else too, Harry.'

'What now?'

'If I'm going to qualify, I need my job back.'

'I thought Morris said your exams weren't under threat?'

'I don't trust them. And there are competencies to do, portfolios. You know how it works.' She sighs. 'And I *need* it, Harry. My job is part of me.'

Harry leans across the worktop, shoulders rounded. '*Fuck.*' The force of his hand hitting the wooden surface makes the bottle rock. 'He was always controlling. You know, once, when he came home from an overnight trip, he realised my mother had rearranged the furniture in the front room. It wasn't how he liked it, so he made her put it all back how it was. He didn't help, he just watched her. When she was done, hot and upset, he kissed her on the cheek and said how nice it was to be home.'

I picture Creighton ordering his wife around and in my imagination his expression is just like it was today. 'Bloody hell, what a creep.'

Harry is full of undirected intensity now and his gaze darts to me. His finger taps subconsciously on the wood of the worktop. 'You know, you could have just declared your love for me and told him to fuck off.' He doesn't wait for an answer. 'You could have done that, couldn't you?'

'We've talked about that.'

'Have we?' He rolls his eyes, then fixes them on me as he drains his glass. His eyes are hooded, his jaw tight. The change in him since talking about his childhood is startling. His eyes have narrowed, taking on a sullen Creighton glare. For a horrible, fleeting moment, he looks exactly like his father. 'So what do we do then?'

Pushing the image aside, I sit beside him. 'I don't know. We need some leverage too. But what can we use? What have we got on them?'

The tension thrums in his arm as I hold it, his eyes fixed on the worktop. He shakes his head, his jaw clenched tight. He is as wired as I've ever seen him.

'I never thought I'd suggest this,' he mutters. 'But why don't we use what happened the other night?'

'How do you mean?'

He won't look at me. 'Morris and Wilson's affair. Wilson is mortified at being discovered. She owes me one now. I think I can persuade her to declare you fit.'

'Are you serious?' My heart leaps at the thought. It's risky, but, if I can get back to work, all Harry and I need to do is pretend to split up for a few months. Then we move away. Start again. We could even apply for jobs abroad afterwards, get away from his family and leave this whole thing behind us. Self-doubt creeps in. 'No, Harry. You're putting your own job at risk.'

'Not if I phrase it right.' Now he looks at me, eyes hard. 'Subtext is everything. She'll get the drift without me needing to spell it out for her.'

He hands me his empty glass silently, wanting a refill. My heart is hammering with excitement at the chance of working again. I'm halfway through filling the glasses at the worktop when I sense Harry close behind me. As I turn to hand him his glass, he grips my hand against it. My fingers are turning white with the pressure of his hand on mine. Pain shoots through my knuckles. 'Harry, you'll break it.'

The grip loosens, just enough for a little blood to rush back into my fingers. He takes the glass from me but stays close. His eyes are filled with anger, cobalt grey like a night sea. He takes a sip, his gaze fixed on mine. At waist level, his fist is clenched. He notices me staring at it and his hand relaxes.

'I'm sorry. But I can't tell you how much that manipulative bastard winds me up, Edie.'

'Yeah, clearly,' I manage quietly, breathing too fast. My mouth is dry.

The thunder in his eyes lingers, flickering. Then he returns to his seat at the breakfast bar, the tension in his body finally loosening. He puffs his cheeks. 'I'm so sorry, I don't know what came over me. It's just *him*, that's all. Not you. This is all down to him.'

'Yeah.'

'I love you.'

'I know you do.' A little louder this time.

'So I'll give this a try, for you. I won't say anything about it.' He looks up again. 'And I'll think of what I can say to Wilson to get you back to work. Okay?'

'Okay.' My glass clinks against my teeth. My previous thought is echoing through my consciousness: *he looks like his father.*

Harry has inherited wealth, status, privilege – and okay, good looks – from James Creighton, and I thought that was where the similarities ended. I have only ever seen the boyish Harry, have only ever witnessed the loving, sensitive side.

But what if other things are inherited too, darker things? Things learned, ingrained.

They say the apple never falls far from the tree.

What if that's a little too close for comfort?

29

Edie

The truth feels harder in the cold light of morning, Harry's anger somehow less threatening. Nothing more is said, and he sits on the bed in silence as I pack. We kiss and promise to phone each day, although it feels like the passionless 'going to work' kiss of a thirty-year marriage. But then, in his eyes I see the same Harry I've come to love since the day he waited outside the department to ask me out, like a nervous teenager might. From the door, he watches my car reverse out into the road, then he raises one hand as I leave. My foot hovers over the brake when I see his head drop, hair falling across his forehead, but then it is too late and the door closes. In the car doubt settles over me; why am I doing this to him? To us? I have to keep reminding myself; neither Harry nor I have created this situation. James Creighton sees the problems I'm having as a perfect excuse to get me away from his son. Harry and I are the victims in this.

When I arrive at Jaz's, she's as blunt as ever. 'This is *your* life, honey,' she reminds me, 'and if Harry can't see how important work is to you, then he needs to take a long hard look at himself.'

Jaz's flat is as unconventional as she is; the place is crammed with nick-nacks from various holidays she has been on, framed posters of films, Moroccan throws, Thai wall hangings, and cushions of so many different colours and styles, it's like a festival glamping pod. The bedroom door is ajar, and her bed is unmade. The duvet is ruffled and messed up in a way that only a bed that has recently had two people in it can be.

I nod at the bed and smile. 'Have I interrupted something?'

Her eyes widen, her mouth opens. 'Oh my God, Edie. Are you some kind of detective?'

'No… just asking.'

'Well, he's gone. He left an hour ago.'

'Matt?'

'Maybe.' She pushes me playfully and shakes her head. 'I'm supposed to be asking you the questions.'

She makes us some coffee and we sit down. Jaz confesses that Matt stayed over and tells me about their date. She laughs that it was the sort of date teenagers might go on: bowling, then pizza and beer. So, Matt got his wish after all. Then she becomes more serious.

'When we got back here, we just opened up with each other. We talked for hours. He is more like you and me than I realised, Edie. A deep thinker, and a good listener too. I found myself talking about my problems from years ago. About what I did to myself back then, the depression. How the job turned me around. Even my hopes for the future.'

'This sounds serious, Jaz.'

'I don't know. Maybe. You're the only other person I've opened up to so quickly. It feels right though.' She smiles and puffs her cheeks. 'Anyway, go on, tell me. What happened?'

'Harry's dad is interfering with our relationship. He's been investigating my past, Jaz, can you believe that? It feels horribly invasive.' As the words leave my lips I'm blindsided again by the image of a girl's hair swaying gently in the movement of the tide. She is so still in the water. The image washes over me on a wave of guilt, but that moment in time is all I can reach, and it slides away again. In the pause, Jaz frowns.

'Edie, are you okay?'

'Yeah. Just a… memory.' The image has gone, leaving just a trace. I change the subject, although the guilt remains, like white noise in the background. 'So now I know. Harry's father has been checking up on me. When was it you saw him at the KG again?'

'At the conference. It went on all day at the postgraduate centre. Morris had gone because Amy Wilson was giving a keynote speech.

161

We know how close those two are. Secretly, I think they're having an affair.'

'Those two? You're kidding.' I force a shocked grin, overplaying my surprise. If the affair comes out, Harry and I have lost the one decent card we have in our hand. 'No, he's too uptight. Too clinical.'

Jaz shudders. 'That's probably why we're always short of chlorhexidine scrub; he likes to sterilise everything before he gets down to it.'

'That's disgusting, Jaz. You're sick.' I laugh. 'Go on…the conference?'

'Yeah. To be honest, we wouldn't really have known it was happening if Morris hadn't gone to it. You know how insular it gets in the unit. Anyway, this guy comes back, slick as hell, looking all senior and serious.'

'He's a professor.'

'Right. He looked it. He and Morris stood by Cox's bedside and talked for a while; I didn't hear much. I got your name once or twice though. What's going on, Edie?'

'He wants to split me and Harry up, and we're playing along. Just until I qualify. In the meantime, Harry is going to have a word with Wilson, see if he can persuade her to declare me fit to work.' At Jaz's frown, I shrug. 'Harry knows how desperate I am to qualify in September.'

'So desperate that you'll let him go crawling to Wilson?'

'It was his idea. Work is everything, Jaz – surely you, more than anyone, understand that?'

She's seen the evidence. I stay late, do extra shifts, fighting to be the best trainee the department has. She knows how important it is to me, more than anything else in my life, even Harry. With only Mum's income, things were tight when I was younger. Mum had enough from Dad's life insurance to pay off the mortgage, just enough to keep us going. But that was all, no more luxuries. Mum was an only child, and both sets of grandparents were dead. We had no wider family to rely on; from the moment Dad died, it was us and no one else. No more talk of fee-paying schools; my father was educated privately and had wanted the same thing for me. That chance had gone, and I wonder whether it has something to do with my need to constantly push myself. But Mum had done her best. *It's not where you go, my darling, it's what you do when you're there.* My memories are clear at this stage in my life, painfully clear. I'd tried to fit in at secondary school. But my loneliness and my desperation to belong clung to me like some horrible smell.

'What are you thinking?' Jaz asks.

'Nothing. Just about my father. How different things might have been if he'd lived. I was just wondering what I would have been like if things in life had come easier to me.'

'Insufferable, probably. You'd be like all the rest of the doctors at the KG.'

I laugh dryly, but the thought of my teenage years has made me weary, tired of hiding things all the time. 'Things are coming back to me piece by piece, Jaz. Do you remember Sophie, the other girl in the photo?'

'Yeah, of course. Why?'

'I think she's Samuel Cox's daughter. I think she died, but I want to know for sure. My mother won't say anything. I don't know what memories I can trust.'

Jaz shakes her head. 'Where's your initiative, doctor? Are you aware how easy it is to find out about people?' She gets up and goes into the kitchen. In a few seconds, she is back with her laptop and a bottle of wine. She holds it up. 'Too early?'

We both look at the clock. 12:15. 'Nah. It's afternoon now, Jaz.'

She grins, gets two glasses from a cabinet and unscrews the cap. 'Do you know the number of times I've researched my boyfriends online?'

'Is that ethical?'

'Give me a break. Do you know how many creeps there are out there?'

She opens the laptop and in minutes is on an ancestry site. I pour two small glasses, then move closer, until we are touching hip to hip, my chin resting on her shoulder, as her fingers fly over the keys. She subscribes with a free trial, punching in her debit card details.

'I'll cancel it tomorrow,' she says and winks. She hits the tab for death certificates.

England. Year range 2000 to 2010.

Name: Sophie Cox.

'She would have been born about the same year as me, in ninety-five.'

She enters the details and hits send. Six matches. She scrolls down the ages at the time of death. 20, 87, 64, 17, 92, 70. No children.

'So does that mean she's not dead?'

'Not unless she had a different name,' Jaz explains. 'Or unless it was never reported.'

I think of her, flying across the sand, laughing and splashing in the waves. I see her with Samuel, as he bends down to kiss her wet hair. Would her death have gone unreported?

No, impossible.

'So she didn't drown?'

'What makes you think she drowned?'

I can't tell her about the image that plagues my thoughts. The reason I might have pushed all of this away for so long, the secret that I'm clinging onto. The only way to be sure of what happened is to go back to where it all happened, and this time I'll make sure no one follows me.

30

Harry

I felt so groggy this morning after a night with no sleep, all I could think of was calling in sick. Then guilt got the better of me, and I finally dragged myself out of bed with a groan of resignation. It's only the second night with her gone, but everything felt out of sync as I got ready, from the empty bed I'd been stretched out across diagonally, to the bathroom without shower gel residue everywhere or the smell of her shampoo, to the kitchen, stark and unwelcoming. Everything felt sterile, like a rental property waiting for someone to move in. I couldn't wait to get out of the place, yet as soon as I got into work I couldn't concentrate properly. There were endless MDT meetings in the morning, the administrator had filled my afternoon diary with clinical assessments, and all I could think of was her.

By the time my last functional diagnosis assessment was over at four, my decision had been made. Spending all day asking myself why I was about to do this had produced one unavoidable answer. I want things back to the way they were, and I am prepared to bend my own principles to do it. In a perfect world, I'd turn the clock back two weeks, but as that's impossible I can at least make sure Edie and I have a future together. So at four-thirty, I'd knocked on Wilson's office door and had fielded her look of surprise and four-day-old embarrassment. The conversation had been stilted. We'd talked about case studies without much enthusiasm, realising we were both just a little too polite and slightly too ready to agree with each other. After fifteen minutes, I had brought up the subject of Edie. *She is getting isolated at home, Amy,* I'd said. *I'm incredibly worried about her.* Wilson had nodded, biding her time until she could see how this played out. I'm not a good liar, but I managed to lay it on thick enough for Wilson to begin seeing this in clinical terms. *Edie is brooding*, I continued, *she is turning in on herself with a continual cycle of negative thoughts. She needs the distraction of work. Please reconsider your decision to put her on sick leave, it's doing more harm than good*.

The image of a flustered, post-coital Wilson, a horrified Morris, and my own shocked expression lingered between us, but nothing was mentioned. There was no acknowledgement, and the air was never cleared as we talked. Despite this, the rawness of the memory in both our minds was more than enough to tip the balance. We both knew I was asking a personal favour, and we knew what I was really saying, but Amy Wilson clung onto the fact that I was basing my request upon a clinical consideration of Edie's mental health. In the end, she nodded.

'I understand that dwelling on the situation at home is going to have an adverse effect on her. I'll talk to Doctor Morris…' here, she made a point of not breaking eye contact '… and we'll see if we can come up with a compromise that will suit everyone.'

'And I must also point out, Amy, that I know my father and you are in touch. I would rather nothing was said to him about this discussion. Well, he doesn't need to know *everything*, does he?'

One pencilled eyebrow raised, almost imperceptibly. She understood the subtext. 'Yes, I suppose.'

And, just as I'd assured Edie, all the meaning in mine and Wilson's conversation was in the things we *didn't* say to each other.

Deception doesn't come easily to me, but after speaking to Wilson, the opportunism of the moment seeped into my mood, and it seemed as good a time as any to talk to my father as well. I had no intention of telling him our plans, but I wanted to speak to him, to look in his face and try to find his motives behind those cold grey eyes of his. I wanted to talk about Edie and see how he reacted. In truth, I hadn't wanted to go back to our empty house either, and the drive out to Warwickshire will help get rid of the nasty taste of coercion after my chat with Wilson. My mother is out this evening so my father is home alone, except for their housekeeper, Yolande. So

I'm going to play the heartbroken son, and I'm going to find out for myself how deep this hatred of her runs in his veins.

As I drive, I replay the previous evening. Inside, I cringe at the way I reacted, the way I somehow switched the blame to Edie. The thought I might lose her for good tortures me, because in that split second of anger I *had* lost her and, after she left, the moment felt like a bereavement. In the kitchen as she told me her plans, for a horrible instant I felt used, powerless. My anger came down like a veil. I've seen it in others – in my father – but never in myself. It's uncomfortable when your own psychology isn't obvious to you. My mind drifts to a forensic case study I once reviewed. Episodic dyscontrol syndrome. Sudden rage, in other words. A mousey-looking salesman had beaten his wife to death with a hammer after some minor disagreement. I can still recall the bemused frown on his face as they interviewed him. *But it wasn't me. I can't have done it,* he'd whispered. *Don't you understand how much I love her?* Denial is one of the most powerful instincts we possess.

My parents' rambling farmhouse is on the outskirts of Wootton Wawen, just beyond Henley-in-Arden. Prime Barbour jacket and Range Rover territory. When I arrive, the main house lights are off, and only Yolande's chalet shows any sign of life. My parents assuage their middle-class guilt at having a housekeeper by giving her lots of time off and letting her use a self-contained annexe in the garden. It gives them the sense they don't own her, but it's all a question of perspective. I let myself in to the empty house and switch the lights on, wandering around, letting the oppressive feeling of home sink into me.

My father's study is open; he never locks it. Why would he? My mother has lost interest in him and his career, and Yolande knows not to venture in there. The smell of the room, a mixture of oak furniture and leather-bound books, always brings back memories. It was where he would hold court on school report day, or when I had to tell him how my exams went. His shelves still hold the same books they have for years. Freud, Jung, Rogers, Skinner. A locked glass cabinet is neatly lined with first editions of novels he admires.

He has a rare 1957 signed copy of Ayn Rand's *Atlas Shrugged*, which cost him thousands. As a child I was fascinated by the cover with its strange dystopian sun hanging over a blank, dead railway tunnel. He would show it to me, boast of how much it was worth, then smack my hand when I tried to touch it.

He has obviously been working in here today, because there are several papers strewn across his desk. As if handling delicate manuscripts, I glance through them. They are mostly reports, committee minutes and other things too boring for words. But in the low light of the green wall lamps, a name has jumped from the mass of papers and typed pages, a letterhead sticking out from a wallet file buried beneath the pile of correspondence. My breathing shallows, as if my breath will somehow trigger him to appear.

Claydon Manor.

Gingerly, I open the file. I scan inside; the letterhead is of a private company that owns Claydon Manor. Steeple Healthcare, a subsidiary of Valhalla Private Equity. *May we reiterate how delighted we are to have you join our senior management team…* I skim further.

… may I also confirm that, following our recent discussion, we would be happy for you to have clinical input at Claydon Manor, and be involved in some of our cases.

I pause, heart hammering. An image of Edie's mother, sitting at the window in a medicated haze, staring out at the landscape, flashes into my mind.

Your experience and knowledge can only add to our already growing reputation for excellence. Our partnership with the NHS Trust is already…

I put the letter down. There's more here, so much more. I scan the papers in the file, pick one up.

A newspaper report, printed from the internet. Edie's case. It's a report I'd read online. I look beneath; further reports. Images.

Shit.

There are sheaves of printouts, clippings. Articles on traumatic repression, dissociative amnesia. It's the work of a meticulous mind, of a born researcher. A collector. There are pages of reports on the abduction, written notes. She's been right about him all along. If she won't face her own past, he is going to discover it for her. Knowledge is power.

A sharp noise pulls my attention from the papers to the hallway outside.

I drop the file back on the desk, slide it under the others. The front door has snapped shut and the kitchen light has clicked on. How did I not hear his car pull up? The drive to the house is gravel; I should have heard him coming.

'Hello?' Then, louder. 'Is that you, Harry?'

I slip out into the hallway, and meet him as he is coming out of the kitchen. He is dressed casually for once; jeans and a sweater. He seems ruffled, breathless. 'When did you get here?'

'Just now, I was looking for you.'

'Ah. I just nipped out.' He turns back to the kitchen. 'You should have called to say you were coming.'

'Well, something happened, and I wanted to tell you in person.'

He flicks the coffee maker on and reaches for a sachet from the cupboard, his composure quickly returning. 'Do you want a coffee?'

'No, thanks.'

'What is it then? What have you got to tell me?'

He's better at this than me, way better. From being surprised, he is now back in control. I sit at the wide island. Here goes. 'Dad, Edie doesn't want to see me any more.'

He doesn't reply, but continues working silently, methodically. Fitting the sachet, starting the machine, getting the mug ready. When this is all done, he speaks. 'I'm so sorry to hear that, Harry. I know how much you liked her. What happened?'

Bravo, a masterful performance. I shrug, trying to look upset. 'I don't know. She finished with me two nights ago. She said, in her exact words, that she no longer loved me.'

He turns, holding his steaming cup. 'You're better off without her then.'

'She's already moved out. She's gone to a friend's house.'

169

'Has she?' His eyebrows arch, and his lips purse in the closest thing he can get to sympathy. 'I hate to ask this, Harry, but there wasn't anyone else involved, was there?'

'I don't know. Maybe.'

'Do you want to talk about it?'

I rest my forehead on my hands for effect, because I don't trust my own performance.

'No, I just wanted to let you know. I don't know what I did wrong.'

He leans on the island. 'Maybe you did nothing wrong? These things happen.'

'Yeah.' I nod without meeting his gaze. 'Be honest though, Dad – you never really liked her, did you?'

He sighs, running a hand though his hair. 'Your mother and I liked Edie a lot, Harry. I don't know what gave you the impression we didn't.'

'You never liked her in the same way you did Nicky.'

'She's different to Nicky, that's all.' He shakes his head, as though I'm being wilfully stupid. 'Name me one time when we ever did anything against her?'

Lies, lies, lies. My loathing towards him becomes almost physical. It lodges in my throat and that's where it stays, desperate to get out. The anger and injustice buzzes like some angry wasp in a bottle. It's at times like this that Freud never seemed more intuitive; sons *do* want to kill their fathers. They're supposed to grow out of it. I clearly haven't. I stare at him as he stirs the cup. My voice sounds steady to my own ears; but if an undercurrent of rage sours it, I couldn't care less.

'You're a lying bastard. You wanted her out of my life from the start.'

He turns. 'What did you say to me?'

'I said you're a lying bastard.'

Then in three long strides, he's across the kitchen and on me, standing face to face. He is two inches shorter than me, but I am now the child. Always the child. I break eye contact. 'You think I didn't like her? Why not tell me earlier then? Why not stand up to me? I'll tell you why, it's because you're weak. And where your welfare is concerned, Harry, I'm right. I've *always* been right.'

'No. This time you're wrong.' My voice hits a fragile, high note. My eyes sting with tears and my cheeks flush with shame. So much for keeping my composure.

He notices. 'Get yourself under control. It's pathetic.'

A female voice tears us away from each other. In the doorway is Yolande, wide-eyed, in loose joggers and hoodie, her hair pulled back. A loaded look passes between her and my father.

'Is everything okay, Mr Creighton? I forgot my phone charger, and I heard voices.'

He steps away, his breathing slowing, his composure returning. He nods curtly, but is not looking at her. 'Yes, everything is fine, thank you, Yolande.'

I'm left shaking, caught between fear and rage, as he walks back to the worktop. As Yolande leaves the kitchen, her worried eyes linger on my father, then wander to me, and I see what's in them. The look she gave him was more than that of housekeeper to employer. Now I know why I didn't hear his car; he was in her chalet with her. More deceit. My heart goes out to my mother and any final thread of respect for him snaps.

'Thanks for the chat, *Dad*.'

'Harry—'

He grabs my arm and I turn on him. 'I hope you're happy now Edie and I are through. I hope you're glad that it's over with the one person I've ever loved. Finished.' I lean down until our faces are nearly touching. 'And just to make it clear, so are you and I.'

'Harry, stop. You're upset. I shouldn't have said those things to you.' As I stride along the hallway toward the front door, he follows. 'Let me explain.'

I stop at the door and turn to face him. 'You want to explain? Then write me a fucking letter, because we're done. From now on, I want you out of my life. I'm not answering your calls, and I don't want you at the house.'

And then the door is shut and I'm crunching across the gravel towards my car, wiping my face angrily where the cool air has found my wet cheeks. I don't look back as I drive away, away from the family home. I'm finished with them both.

As I drive, I put my phone on speaker and scroll through my contacts until I find Edie's number. The visit served its purpose, and at least I know where I stand.

It's me and her now, against him.

31

Edie

I left Jaz's flat at 6 a.m., as the sun crept over the rooftops of Edgbaston, the traffic just starting to gather on the roads. I cleared the industrial units and shopping parks of the outskirts of the city by six-twenty, heading towards the M5, Harry's words echoing in my head. He called me last night, his voice thick with anger, disbelief and frustration, emotions tumbling over each other. His sentences spilled out; fast, urgent, and, as I drove, they tore at me as they did when he first said them. I'd barely had a chance to say hello when he'd dropped the bombshell.

'Edie, my father has a file on you.'

'What?' I'd managed.

'Newspaper reports, clippings.'

The thought makes me feel just as nauseous now as it did then, still forces the same rising wave of bitterness into my throat.

'He has copies of your GMC registration, your CV,' Harry continued. 'There are maps of the coast where Cox took you; even the route of the abduction is marked. Jesus. He must have been down there himself, asking questions about you. Edie, he has your whole history.'

Until then, my suspicions still had the quality of a conspiracy theory: it was possible to dismiss them. But now they've snapped into the crisp focus of hard reality. James Creighton knows everything about me. Probably more than I know about myself.

For the rest of the night I'd stared into the darkness, numb. Then at five, I'd got up and dressed. I'd started driving south towards the coast, with no plan other than to ask people – anyone I could find

– what they knew about the abduction, to discover what he might have found out. But another part of me also wanted to get away from the city, away from him. I wanted time to think. Harry's chat with Wilson had worked; Morris had rung me the day before to arrange a meeting. In hindsight, he'd told me, perhaps we were hasty. I might be better off in a phased return to work in theatres. It's not healthy to be isolated, he said, as if the idea had been his and not Wilson's.

But I need to know what Creighton knows, and everything follows from what happened at the coast. Everything is connected to my relationship with Samuel Cox. I know he is innocent, and that it was my father who abused me, though getting anyone else to believe that is another matter. The fragmented memories of the coast, and of my time there, are not traumatic. But there is one image that is: a single horrible vision of a drowned girl. That one awful feeling of guilt. Cox's daughter is dead, Melanie Cox confirmed that. It has to be linked; it can't be a coincidence. And it's from that final image of Sophie that my dissociation springs, I'm certain of it. The knowledge of what happened to her is what I've been running away from all this time. If she's alive, would anyone be able to find her? And if she drowned, is she traceable? As I was passing the Bristol Channel at Portishead with all of these thoughts swirling around, it came to me. I realised who would have records of drowning incidents along that coastline.

The lifeboat station at Minehead is large and newly built, hiding along a small road at the far end of the harbour, in the shadow of North Hill. This part of the town, far away from the amusement arcades and the souvenir shops, is quiet and green, and the stepped hill that leads up towards Exmoor is blanketed with oaks, cedars and poplars. I arrive mid-morning, Where the station faces the sea, two men and a woman are checking equipment on the lifeboat, which they have pulled out from the docking bay and onto the upper level of the ramp. The female crewmember spots me first. She is about my age, the personification of a surfer girl, with sun-blonde hair and tan.

Her Somerset accent carries down to me. 'Morning. Are you all right there?'

The men have stopped working and are watching me as well. Both are around thirty, the one nearest with a hipster beard and cap pushed back on his head, and the other with close-cropped hair and wraparound sunglasses. All three look like an organic part of the boat, as if they'd be out of place on land.

'Morning,' I reply, squinting up at them. 'I wonder if there is anyone who could help me with some information.'

'What type of information?' The bearded guy's accent is neutral, his tone a mixture of curiosity and suspicion.

'Information on a young girl. She might have drowned off the coast a few years ago.'

'Might have? Don't you know one way or the other?'

I shield my eyes. 'No. I know that sounds odd.'

'If she drowned it'll be in the newspapers.' The guy in the sunglasses repositions a row of lifejackets, and gazes down at me.

'Yes, but it isn't. Look, I know you guys keep records. I'm just trying to cover every base, that's all.'

'Whatever information we have is confidential.'

I hold up my ID badge, appealing hopefully to some mutual respect between the services. 'I'm an ICU doctor. It's patient related.'

They fall silent, glancing at each other. Finally, the bearded guy smiles, giving my badge a cursory glance from the boat. From that distance, I could have been holding up anything. 'Yeah, all right. Maybe I can check our log.'

He climbs down. He is tall and wiry, his skin salt tanned. The clinical side of me assesses the wrinkles that frame his eyes; by the time he is forty, he is going to look sixty. I was wrong about him being out of place on land; he moves with as much lithe self-assurance as he did when he was on the boat. He beckons me into the boathouse.

'My dad was a doctor too,' he says, leading me into the office. 'Wanted me to follow in his footsteps.'

'They always do.'

'Yeah, well, I just wanted to do my own thing. So now I'm a beach lifeguard. As well as doing this on the side.'

'What do you do in the winter?'

'I fuck off somewhere warm.' He puts his hand out. 'I'm Jed, by the way.'

His grip is firm. 'Thanks for doing this, Jed.'

'No problem. So what was the name?'

'Sophie…' I pause on the surname. This next bit is guesswork. 'Sophie Cox.'

'Drowning? What year?'

I hesitate again. It wasn't the summer of the photograph, it was later. When does my memory become clearer? 'Two thousand and seven or two thousand and eight, I think.'

'You think? Okay, it's a start. What month?'

'I don't know.' I pout vaguely at his interrogative gaze. 'Summer, though.'

Jed pulls some files down from a cabinet. He grins at me. 'At least it was back in the days when there was still such a thing as paperwork.' He rifles through a folder. I wait as the pages turn and he reads from each sheet. Finally, he shakes his head.

'Nope. Sorry. No callouts from this station to anyone with the name Sophie Cox. No confirmed deaths at all either summer.' He shrugs apologetically. 'Did she definitely drown?'

'I can't say for sure, I just know…' I hesitate. 'Well, I assumed she drowned.'

'Are you sure the surname is Cox?' An older man, who up until then has been poring over some paperwork, has swivelled his chair and is looking at Jed and me with bright, pale-blue eyes. 'And not Cullen?'

'What are you on about, Bill?' Jed asks, with an apologetic frown.

'Summer? Two thousand and eight? A girl went missing nearby and we did a search for her. Never found anything though.'

Jed slaps Bill on the shoulder. 'Bill was born a few miles up the coast; he's about as inbred as they come,' he explains. 'Right, Bill?'

Bill treats Jed to an expression of withering contempt. 'You need to learn some respect, Jed. The girl was called Sophie. Sophie Cullen. A girl from the local care home. We did a search of the area after it was reported. It's all in the notes.'

Jed furrows his brow at the folder. 'Yeah, you're right. Sophie

Cullen. Reported missing on the twentieth July two thousand and eight. The police asked us to check the coastline just in case.'

'So she was reported missing, not drowned?'

'Yeah. By a friend she was with on the beach.'

'A friend? Can I ask who?'

'Yeah, I guess.' He scans the sheet again, but I already know what's coming. 'I've only got the surname. Carter.'

So I was there that day. I reported her missing, not drowned. But the memory of Sophie in the sea is real, unbearably real. I fish the photograph from my bag and hold it out to Bill, my heart hammering as he looks at it. 'Do you recognise the girl?'

He studies it for several seconds, which feel like hours. 'Yeah, maybe. I don't know. When was this taken?'

'Two thousand and three. She would have been about eight then.'

'The girl who went missing was eleven or twelve, so it would fit. But it does prove one thing, love.'

'What?' I ask.

Bill's eyes narrow as he hands the photograph back. 'It proves you were lying about why you're here. This isn't to do with a bloody patient. That other girl in the photo is you, isn't it?'

'I'm sorry,' I reply, breathing too heavily as my pulse gradually slows. 'Yes, Sophie was... well, it's personal.'

He studies me for a moment, then pulls the file across and reads it. 'Okay, I suppose it's no secret. It was even in the local paper. We checked the coast from Watchet to Porlock Weir, but she wasn't found.'

'Yeah, but that doesn't mean she didn't drown,' Jed chips in. 'If she drowned up-channel from here, she'd go under for a couple of days. The tide would pull her along. This is an estuary, you see,' he tells me before turning back to the others. 'So by the time she surfaced again, she might be a few miles out. Then she's gone for good.'

Out past the windows that face onto the harbour, the wide channel rolls along. In the far distance, a faint grey line marks the Welsh coast. But the scenery is background to what I am really seeing. Long hair waving in the water; she is floating. Not something imagined, something real. This proves it.

I turn to the old man. 'Bill, what care home was it?'

'The Elms near Willerton. But it's closed now.'

'Who could I ask about the missing girl then?'

'Check around the town. The older folk might remember the case, but I doubt it.'

I thank them and leave, but before the door has closed they've already gone back to their morbid discussion about the tides, and how far a body might be rolled along to the sea, and where Sophie Cullen's bones might now lie.

After several hours of walking around Willerton, knocking on doors and showing the photo, my feet are aching and my head throbs. Even the older residents I asked were vague. Yes, they said, they remembered the case. A young girl did go missing from the care home years ago, but they had forgotten her name until I reminded them. It didn't even make the local news for long; the care home was in special measures, they said, Sophie wasn't the first person to run away. She was young, but so were the others. They were troubled, and many had problems with drugs and alcohol.

In a cafe on Willerton High Street, my coffee goes cold as I search the internet for her. The photo they had used for the appeal was taken at some care home party or similar, cropped to show her face and a portion of the background. The shoulders of other unseen people at the table touch hers, and she is staring at the camera resentfully. Her hand hovers near her forced half-smile as if she wants to cover her mouth. Braces glint awkwardly between her lips. She is alone in the crowd, as if she's hating every second of it. She is as isolated as a young girl can be, and my throat tightens with compassion.

I look at the picture. There is no question they are the same girl. Anyone could see it.

The cafe owner, a woman in her late sixties in a floral pinafore, comes to take my half-finished coffee away. She smiles, and I imagine her starved for conversation in these quiet out-of-season months. I smile back briefly, not wanting to talk, and my eyes drift back to my phone screen.

'Why all the sudden interest in Sophie Cullen?' I hear her say behind me. She is looking over my shoulder at the screen.

'Pardon?' I ask, as politely as I can, laying my phone face-down.

'Sophie. That girl who went missing?'

'Did you know her?'

'Not directly. I just heard of the case years ago.' She puts the cup on the counter, talking over her shoulder. 'I couldn't tell that other person much about her either.'

'What other person?'

'The man that was asking about her, a week or two back. Older guy. Very distinguished fellow, he was, if you like that sort of thing.' She laughs. 'A real silver fox.' She notices my expression and comes across to the table. 'I'm sorry, I didn't mean to speak out of turn. I just wondered about the sudden interest in the girl. Was she a relative?'

'No.'

My hands are trembling as I fumble a five-pound note from my pocket and drop it on the table. My legs just about support me as I get up to leave, her eyes following me. 'That's too much, love,' she calls after me, but I'm already outside.

My thoughts are running away from me, slipping out of reach, just as my old, safe life seems to be. Creighton is ahead of me; he knows what happened to Sophie already. The only people who knew about her were me, Harry and my mother. Harry wouldn't say anything to his father about the photo, would he? No. He's on my side, I'm certain of it. Which means only one thing. I think of that long dark hair swaying in the water, floating, lifeless. And me staring, motionless. I think of the guilt, and everything I've blocked out since them. But I know what caused the trauma now. And I think of my mother, heavily medicated, pliable, vulnerable.

She has talked about what happened. I watched Sophie drown. I let it happen. Why didn't I help? The memories may be vague, but the guilt is real and intense enough to make me drag deep lungfuls of air in to fight the nausea rising from my core.

Harry's father has finally got to her. And now he knows too.

32

Samuel Cox

There is a hum of conversation in the distance, just murmurs. Someone laughs out loud; a high, spontaneous sound, which feels out of place against the muted noise of the ICU machines. Some private joke amongst the nurses. The laughter fades as time slips again, and the machines become quiet. He follows wherever his mind takes him, wandering along overgrown paths into the past. He hears laughter again, but now it is a child's voice. An eight-year-old's laugh, clear and happy.

They are playing on the beach, a hundred yards from where he is sitting. The sun feels hot on his back, and he reaches into the bag for the bottle, which is helping to soothe his pounding head. He squints at the glare coming from the sea and watches them run across the sand. They find something interesting and bend down to look at it, Edie pointing at the floor, showing whatever she's seen to Sophie. But their attention soon wanders, and they begin running again, this time towards the sea. Edie is last in, careful, cautious. Sophie splashes her gently and soon they are both in together, waving back at him. Playing. Their screams reach him faintly.

The white light of the sun on the sea shimmers and oscillates, like the memory. He drifts again, remembering how Edie had found Sophie playing alone, had made friends with her. Sophie had said she was with a group who had come to the beach for the day but hadn't wanted to say anything more. Edie was shy and reserved with other children even before then. He should have seen it sooner; he should have seen the change in her personality earlier. Even then she was showing signs of what Michael was doing to her. But Sophie had brought out the best in her, and now the girls had taken themselves off together and were inseparable. Perhaps Edie had seen in Sophie someone who was just as scared as she was.

Did he neglect Edie in favour of Sophie that summer? He looked at Sophie and was flooded with love, and he had tried to give her back something he felt she was lacking. He had seen in her something he knew from his own childhood. Loneliness. And she warmed to him, too. On the first day, she ran to him showing where her hand was running with blood. *I cut it on a rock, Sam*, she told him, and he'd dressed the bleeding thumbnail for her, that one caring act enough for the bond to be sealed forever. He swung her highest whenever she ran to him, as Edie watched. It became an obsession with him for the week; whenever she would come to the beach with the people from the home, he would make her day as pleasant as it could be, and he would treat her as if she were his own. He had a wife and daughter already, but there was something in this thrown-together family that felt more genuine. During his one-week holiday here, he would find excuses to go off alone; partly to drink, but also just to be with the two girls. He and Jenny were still talking then, but the end of their friendship was in sight. He knew the fact that he was beginning to suspect what her husband was doing was driving a wedge in between them all.

But he didn't know that it would come to a dramatic head only eleven months later.

As he drifts, the memories slip through his grasp again. For a moment, in the half-world he is existing in, the warmth of that summer is as real to him now as it ever was. But by degrees, the sounds of the hospital intrude, softly, but enough to make the vision begin to fragment and separate.

Edie, I loved you. I still love you.

Didn't I prove that by what I did?

Please tell me you don't believe the lies in the newspapers. They all turned against me, everyone. Please tell me you were still on my side, even then.

The other memories of the coast are harder, and they are pushing through the fog now. They are of the time he took her away, desperate, lost. Unsure of what else to do. He knew it couldn't last, and he knew that he was never going to be believed when he said he did it for her. He knew they would find them soon.

That final night together, just before they came to get Edie, was cold, and the stars were brittle and sharp in the sky. He had sat and watched her sleeping, understanding, in a profound, unbearable flash of pain, that he would never see her as a child again.

I couldn't save you from him, Edie. Forgive me.

That knock on the door meant those summer days were over, and he was entering a bitter season of suffering, far worse than anything he'd ever known.

But he never realised it would last as long as it had.

Now, he just wants to see her. One more time.

33

Edie

When I pull up at Claydon Manor it is nearly five o'clock. I've come straight from the coast, ringing Harry on the way. The news that his father had been there before me hadn't surprised him. We'd agreed it wouldn't be a good idea for him to come with me to see my mother in case we're seen together, and it gets back to his father. I take my work lanyard out of the glove box and drape it over my neck, although a University Hospitals Birmingham NHS Trust badge has no jurisdiction here. Still, a badge is a badge, and people tend to respect them. My self-confidence and sense of authority needs all the help it can get.

I already knew before today that I needed to get my mother away from Claydon Manor and out of James Creighton's reach; now, it's become imperative. As soon as Harry told me that his father had been building a file on me, I'd made my mind up that she's not staying. If she doesn't want to be at home, we can find another place for her to get treatment, but I'm getting her out of there. I don't want to have to face Willard, particularly considering what I'm about to do, so I'm relieved to find out she's not on shift. The nurse in charge is a guy in his mid-forties called Stefan, shuffling around the lobby in civvies, with a small enamel name badge the only thing distinguishing him from one of his clients.

When I approach, he smooths his greying ponytail back and looks me up and down suspiciously. There is a small spot of unidentifiable food decorating the front of his creased shirt. In terms of effort versus reward, ironing your clothes has to be up there somewhere.

The only part of Stefan's shirt not creased is the part that stretches across his beer belly.

His personality seems as easy-going and flexible as his grooming regime, the polar opposite to Sue Willard. When I explain who I am, and that I'm here to see Jenny Carter, he nods and waves me through, glancing briefly at my badge.

'Normally you're supposed to call us first, Doctor Carter. I'll let you through, though. Your mother is in the main unit day room.'

'Thanks,' I reply to the stain on his shirt. Then, as an afterthought. 'Could you let me know what medication my mother is currently on please? I did ask her, but she gets confused.'

'Well…'

I force some authority into my voice. 'I'm a doctor, Stefan. And presumably family members have a right to know what medication their loved ones are prescribed?'

'Sure. Sorry.' He shrugs. 'I'll write it down and bring it in.'

If it wasn't for the fact she is in the day room rather than her bedroom, I would swear that my mother hadn't moved since I last saw her. Her position in her chair is fixed, staring. For years, she has been on what Harry sometimes calls the elastic band pathway; she becomes an inpatient for a few months, and she stabilises, her medication is assessed and corrected where needed, then she goes home again. Permanently bouncing back and forth. In here, her mood swings flatten out, like great waves slowly decreasing into small ripples. In her lowest troughs of depression, she occasionally has Electro-Convulsive Shock therapy. Yes, they still do that. But no matter what her treatment regime, she has always been free to leave, and now it's my job to persuade her to do exactly that.

As soon as I see her, I know she is heavily medicated. Her watery eyes take a moment to adjust, to focus and recognise me. There is a fleeting frown as she searches her memory, and then the shadow of a smile reaches her lips. I sit down and take her hand. They must have increased her dose of sedative. Her dull grey eyes meet mine and a sharp stab of anger pierces me.

'Christ, what have they given you?'

She looks away, scans the floor. 'Edie, I'm so tired.'

'Mum, I know what happened at the coast. Sophie's dead, isn't she? I was there, I saw it happen. Was I to blame? Were you protecting me? I'll understand.'

'You'll understand? How generous.'

'And I know it was Dad who abused me. Don't deny it any more.'

She laughs, a low rattle. A fragile ripple of air. Her finger forms a hook, and she gently touches my head, tapping my temple. 'You think you know everything, don't you? It's all in there. We're all hiding things. So many secrets.'

'Look, Dad's dead. It's okay. I just need you to tell me everything, because you've been speaking to James Creighton, haven't you? What does he know?'

She mimics my voice, taunting. Her voice is high and querulous. 'Look, Dad's dead.'

'For God's sake, Mum. Please.'

Her voice is now a conspiratorial slur. 'He didn't have a heart attack, you know.'

'My father?'

'Michael. It wasn't his heart. I lied about that too.'

'What do you mean?'

But all she does is laugh softly to herself. She hasn't looked at me once since I came in. We are broken apart, her and me, and there is no one who can put us back together again. For years, I'd hoped there would still be the chance that one day we'd be able to love each other like we used to years ago. Looking at her now, I finally realise the chance has gone. We will never be like we were. The secrets that held us together, the feeling of me and her against the world, are cracking apart. Finally, she looks and there are tears in her eyes.

'They believed he took his own life. The suicide of a devastated father. But they were wrong.'

'Mum, what are you saying?'

'He was drunk. Almost passed out. It was easy.'

Her words are spiralling into a place I don't want to go because once this is out, there is no putting it back. His face materialises in my mind again. Michael Carter; that vague figure from family photos and holiday snaps. Michael Carter, the abuser. The man who wrecked the life of this broken woman in front of me. There was no forgetting for *her*. No blank spaces. She may not have spoken about it, but she has carried this for the last two decades.

'They were *my* sleeping tablets, you see,' she continues. 'I crushed them up, managed to make him drink them. I made sure he kept them down. Then I sat and watched him die.' Her eyes struggle to focus on me. But I have misread the tears. They are not tears of guilt, or sorrow. This is no *mea culpa*; it is a declaration of victory. It is exultation, satisfaction. 'Don't you see? It was justice for what he'd done to my lovely girl. To me.'

As she turns back to the window, I am numb. Emotionless. It's impossible to believe this frail woman was capable of such calculated revenge. Her own form of personal retribution. But it's all there in her eyes, in that one moment before the fog descends again. How could she have kept it a secret for so long? How did she keep that locked away, living with knowing she would kill her husband rather than tell the truth? Murder him rather than admit she knew what was happening to her daughter.

She is capable of murder. Exactly how similar are we?

'Mum, have you told James Creighton this?'

Her eyes are glazed again, as if the revelation never happened. 'I don't remember.'

'What have you told him about Sophie? Did she drown?'

She reaches out and holds my sleeve, leaning towards me. 'You tell me.' She lets me go and slumps back in her chair.

'I'm getting you out of here. Come on, let's go.'

I try to help her stand, but she is a dead weight, and her legs don't support her. She shouts, pulling her hand away; her voice echoes around the day room.

'Leave me alone.'

As she falls back into her chair again, the door opens and Stefan shambles in. In his hand he has some paperwork. He gazes across at the two of us and holds the file up.

'Your notes. Is everything okay, Doctor Carter?'

'Why is my mother in this condition, Stefan? Why is she so lethargic?'

His brow furrows. 'I only came on this morning, but in the handover they said she hadn't slept for days. She's been having Trazodone to help.'

'Trazodone along with the antidepressants? For God's sake, what are you playing at?'

'Er, I'm sorry, I haven't…' He reaches for the file again. 'I've got your mother's medication details here if you want to have a look.'

I scan the medication. Diazepam 5mg twice daily. Trazodone, 75mg daily. As well as her SSRIs. No wonder she can barely function. I'm about to drop the file on the table in disgust when a thought occurs. I scan across to the signature of the prescriber. It's hard to read, but yes, it could be. It is a scribbled, slanting scrawl, but I can make out the J and the C.

James Creighton.

Heart pounding, I flip the notes, skimming through to see what has been written about her. I skim faster, pretending not to notice as Stefan inches closer, his discomfort at letting me see the notes palpable. In the corner of my eye his hand reaches out, wanting the file back. His face wears the half-smile of someone who thinks he has made a mistake but isn't sure how to correct it.

'Actually, I don't think you should really be looking at those without permission, Doctor Carter,' he ventures.

Now the firmness in my voice isn't an act. I meet his gaze. 'It's my mother, I'll do what I think is best for her.'

He doesn't reply and I continue to flip through. I take my phone out, planning to photograph the medication page. This is proof that James Creighton has overstepped the mark. Evidence of misconduct. She is not psychotic; she doesn't need this level of medication. I've got him. I flip back, trying to keep my composure, but, as the pages skim beneath my thumb, the notes are snatched out of my hand. Stefan glares at me, closing the file, his easy-going, shabby manner gone. For the first time, I notice the broadness of his shoulders, his posture, the attitude that suggests he's no stranger to confrontation. His stance is wide, his mouth a tight slit. The affable smile has been replaced by a cold stare.

'I said, you're going to need permission.'

My resolve wavers, and I'm scrabbling against the cold, sheer wall of my own low self-esteem. I'm senior to this man, but I'm slipping backwards, into the passivity that I've been kicking against for years. I meet his eyes, and I dare him to interfere as I bend to slip my arms around my mother's bird-like chest.

'Come on, Mum. I'm going to take you home.' I try standing her again, speaking over my shoulder to Stefan. 'I'll tell you what's going to happen, shall I? I'm going to put her in another unit. She hates this place. I want her to be somewhere else.'

'Doctor Carter, you can't do that.'

'Just get a wheelchair for her, Stefan, or I'll fucking report you.'

His hand encircles my forearm. Not gripping hard yet, but firm enough to show me his strength. 'I said you can't take her away.'

'You just watch me.'

'You can't take her.' His hand tightens now, and his voice has flipped into a hard, uncompromising growl. 'Because she's under a Section Three.'

'What?' I swivel. Section Three, involuntary admission up to six months with a final review. Possibility to extend indefinitely. She's here as long as they want her. The main unit day room, he'd said. A polite way of saying the secure unit. 'Who did that without consulting me?'

'I don't know without checking. But I do know that you can't take her with you.'

He may not know who sectioned her, but I do. Stefan and I are facing each other, but it's me who is breathing hard, flushed and close to tears. Stefan is immoveable, implacable. My mother is staring out of the window again, oblivious to what's happening around her.

I turn to her, desperate. 'Mum, please. Come on, let's go.'

Stefan moves closer. 'Doctor Carter, let's not turn this into a problem for security to deal with. I'll get help to remove you if I need to.' In the light from the window, his shadow is between us. 'You can ask for an appointment with her clinician, Doctor Murray. She will explain everything.'

'Murray? James Creighton is running this show, Stefan. Stop lying to me.'

'Please. I think you should go now.' Stefan's arm appears between us, helping me to stand, guiding me away.

'You made her this way. I'm going to report this,' I shrug his hand off. But as he steps backwards, shaking his head, I feel her touch on my arm. My mother is holding my wrist gently, almost lovingly, and she is staring into my eyes. She guides me closer.

'Come here.'

Wary, I lean in, and then I can feel her cheek against mine and a soft kiss on my cheek. Her voice is a whisper. 'You know what you did, my girl.'

'No,' I whisper. 'I don't remember.'

'Yes, you do. It's time to remember. Just like I do.'

'No, Mum. Please.' Her fingers are laced around my wrist, her free hand is on the back of my neck, holding me gently, yet pulling me close with surprising strength every time I try to pull away. I don't want to hear what she has to say. I don't want to know.

'Yes, my darling. It's time to face it.'

'No.'

But then she talks, whispers into my ear, and I can't pull away. I can't escape. She holds me gently like she used to do when I was younger, when I was scared. When all of those hidden monsters rose up from the darkness, and I couldn't look at them for fear of going mad. Except now she is on their side. Now she is making me look. Now she is turning my face to see them, holding me. She talks, her voice a low hiss, and she tells me everything, as the tears run down my cheeks and onto hers.

How did we manage to cope for so long, Mum? How did we?

As the words spill from her lips, as the truth tears me down and everything crumbles, a well begins rising unstoppably inside me, a surge, a floodtide, threatening to wash me away completely. She rips apart the veil of denial I've been hiding behind for so many years, and as she speaks I know every word she says is true.

Then I can hear a noise, building and growing, its pitch steadily increasing. A noise suitable to this kind of place. It's a scream, a yell of pure grief, and it's coming from me. I pull away from her, tear myself away from her grip, standing up on fragile, shaking legs, which threaten to give way any moment.

'No, you're wrong,' I yell. She smiles sadly and shakes her head, the fresh tears on her face mixing with mine. I point an accusatory finger towards her. 'You're lying'

'Doctor Carter, you'd better calm down.' I'd forgotten Stefan was even there. He was too far away to hear what she said, but not too far to see that I'm shaking uncontrollably.

'Don't tell me to calm down,' I hiss. 'You're the ones who got her in this fucking state.'

My anger is raw, edging towards panic. Stefan steps closer. Then, in a moment of clarity, the situation sinks in. The blind fear, the raging guilt, my mother's accusation. Everything coalesces and then something inside of me breaks. I can almost hear it snap, and a sudden sense of immense calm descends on me. A warm feeling of being back in control. What does it matter what I did in the past? What does it change, here and now? I become acutely aware of how my outburst must look, and I force myself to get on top of my rage. Before my mother hissed lies into my ear, I was already starting to sound unbalanced against Stefan's measured, firm tone. Now, if anyone were watching this objectively, they would see a young woman, her eyes red, tired, tear-filled, becoming increasingly agitated in an institution where hysterical is the worst possible thing you can be. Taking several long, deep breaths, I dare Stefan to escalate this further. He doesn't, but neither does his expression mellow.

I turn to my mother, not caring what Stefan hears any more. 'I'm coming back for you, Mum. I love you.'

Then I brush past Stefan as I leave. He glances at my mother, before stalking after me with the determined stride of a man who is about to report everything he has just seen.

34
Edie

By Monday and my first day back at the hospital, the emotional visit to my mother has faded into its true context. I can rationalise her wild allegations. She was heavily medicated, her mind drifting between clarity and confusion. I need to look at anything she says in that place with the cocktail of sedatives they have her on in mind, and take her accusations with a pinch of salt. The past gets mixed up in her mind, which is what worries me because who knows what she's telling Creighton. I'm still desperate to get her out of there, but for now have my first day back at the King George to occupy me. The sense of calm that came over me after my outburst at Claydon Manor still remains. If I lose focus now, I lose everything.

Not surprisingly, Amy Wilson has taken the line of least resistance and stayed away from my morning meeting with Morris. He sits across the desk from me like an interviewer and doesn't look at all embarrassed to see me. For a moment I'm puzzled, then I realise he is blissfully unaware that I know about him and Wilson. I'm not going to enlighten him. Neither am I going to let it show that, where I'm concerned, his authority is crumbling. It's clear now I was wrong about the power dynamics of their relationship. Letting me back to work is a seismic shift in his position, and he has deferred to Wilson. His lover has said the word, and I've flipped from a troubled soul who needs sick leave to a young doctor who's fit to work again. I smile back at him grimly. Why are we so brainwashed to believe in the sanctity of hierarchy? The great Richard Morris is just as flawed, fallible and obviously led by his libido as the next guy.

Even though I was looking forward to coming back to work, that didn't stop me from having a sleepless night thinking about it. Hopefully I'm managing a cooperative expression. Morris starts first.

'Well, Edie. I'm happy to have you back.'

I bite my tongue. We both know how conflicted he really is to see me here. 'Thank you, Doctor Morris. I'm pleased to be working again.'

'I'm also relieved that you are engaging with Amy Wilson again.'

'Well, seeing as you made it a condition of my return.'

He nods, keeping his thoughts to himself, his expression neutral. 'Okay. Well, I have arranged for you to work with Doctor Drake for the week. You'll be on the general surgery list, to get you back into the swing of things. You can start after lunch in theatre four. If you can make sure you're there for twelve-thirty, please, to take part in the afternoon huddle? Please remember, working in ICU is off the table until we have the issue with Mr Cox resolved, in one way or another.'

One way or another? What exactly does he mean by that? Empowered by the knowledge that having me back was down to Wilson's influence, I decide to press him. 'Doctor Morris. I was wondering about Mr Cox. I accept you don't want me involved in his care, and I'm sorry for being so uncooperative about that before, but I'm sure you won't mind me asking about his current condition.'

'He's improving. Extubation looks likely soon, but nothing is ever certain with patients like him. I think that's probably all you need to know right now.'

'Can I ask one more question? If you don't mind?'

'Of course,' he says, still secure in his illusion of power.

'Are you and Amy Wilson friendly with my fiancé's father, Professor Creighton?'

He doesn't miss a beat. He and Wilson have clearly been discussing this. 'Professor Creighton is a good friend of Doctor Wilson's. They have worked together extensively in the past. I have met him too, of course. But I don't see what relevance this has.'

'As I'm sure you'll understand, given my relationship with his son, I would rather Professor Creighton was not made privy to any information shared during my sessions with Amy Wilson from now on. The same goes for my work in general.'

His expression darkens, and he flushes slightly. 'Naturally,' he says firmly. 'Do you think Doctor Wilson and I care nothing for confidentiality?'

I'm within my rights to ask and he knows it, but his fleeting moment of self-doubt has given me all the information I need. Yes, Doctor Morris, sharing information without permission would be unethical. Of course you would say my sessions will remain confidential. With your poker face, you will tell me that James Creighton will never be informed of the personal things I discuss.

But as well as being an adulterer, you're also a terrible liar.

While waiting for my list to start, I spend the morning mooching around the edge of the theatre suite. The ICU at the King George is only forty metres from the entrance to main theatres, so, I can hover between the two without attracting too much suspicion. I spoke to Jaz earlier, and I know she is doing a drugs check this morning, so I'm hoping to speak to her in private. The only time I've ever seen Morris go anywhere the drugs cupboard is when he used it to put me in my place not so long ago.

At about ten, my phone pings. Jaz.

I'm in the cupboard, come and have a chat

I drift out of the theatre staffroom and along the corridor, to where the door to main theatres meets the link corridor. I scan my staff card on the SALTO entry pad and am pleased when the light flashes green. So my card is still working. I bleep myself into ICU; the drug cupboard door is propped open, and Jaz has her back to it, multi-coloured packets of drugs spread out on the counter. She looks up as I close the door behind me.

'Hey. It's good to see you back in scrubs, where you belong. How did the meeting with his lordship go?'

'Okay. It confirmed one thing, as if I didn't know. Creighton is definitely keeping an eye on me. And I'm pretty sure Wilson is still going to pass on information from our meetings to him.'

'I hope you know what you're doing.'

'Not really, Jaz,' I reply. She frowns quizzically at me, so I elaborate. 'Let's just say I'm winging it.'

How do I tell her about my visit to Claydon Manor, about what really happened to Michael? That my mother, for all her apparent delicacy, killed her own husband? Okay, maybe she has flights of fancy under the influence of the drugs they're pumping into her, but I could see in her eyes she meant it. She was practically gloating about it. It was her own particular form of revenge for what he did. Coming so soon after Cox was convicted, it was as if she was determined to stop what was happening for good, there and then. But keeping quiet about it all those years? And never advocating for a man she knew was innocent? What a burden of guilt she has carried.

What's more, how do I express to Jaz the fear that under all that medication she has whispered this secret to James Creighton? For now, all I can do is throw myself into work, because that's the only option I've got. Past the open door, the bays are out of sight, but Samuel Cox's silent presence is still like a magnet.

'Tell me everything about Cox's condition, Jaz. What's he on at the moment?'

'Cox is how you'd expect for someone who is being kept sedated and monitored,' she replies. 'He's on TIVA; propofol and rocuronium. Morris has also diagnosed a small pyogenic liver abscess and has put him on five hundred milligrams of metronidazole every eight hours. He has a morphine pump running at two milligrams per hour to cover any breakthrough pain from the abscess.'

'What about inotropes?'

'No, he's off them.' She pauses. 'Edie, I've got some news. I think Morris is going to have to wake him up on Friday. There have been questions about why he's still intubated.'

My heart hammers, thinking of him sitting up, awake. Talking. 'Questions from who?'

'Everyone. The other consultants, Johnstone, Al-Ghazi, Dacre.

They say the space is needed. They have big cases coming through theatres who are having to go to High Dependency instead of Intensive Care. I don't want him to be extubated, Edie. I'm worried. I don't want to have to treat this guy when he's awake.'

'Why?'

'I don't know, I just don't. Morris has been really off with me recently as well. Somehow, everything that goes wrong is my fault now, as if he's deliberately undermining me. As if he doesn't trust me any more.'

'Everyone trusts you, Jaz.'

'I'm sure Morris doesn't for some reason. Anyway, the last couple of weeks have knocked my confidence, to the point where looking after Samuel Cox when he wakes up scares me.'

'Don't be worried, Jaz, it'll be fine.' I think of Cox waking up and try to keep my voice steady. 'This is something I've been waiting for, for weeks.'

She takes my arm. 'Edie, I've been thinking, do you really want to speak to this guy? Seriously, what's wrong with letting Morris take the heat off you a little? He's a prick, but why not keep your head down and let him deal with it?'

'We've talked about this, Jaz. I just don't like the feeling they're all in it together, that's all.'

She sighs loudly, puffing her cheeks. 'I know I'm in a weird place right now as well, but seriously, Edie, you see conspiracies where there aren't any.'

'You don't know what I know, Jaz.' At her puzzled look, I start getting drugs down from the cupboards. 'Come on, let me help you with this check.'

Reluctantly, she lets me; I call out the name of the drug and count out the quantities we have, while she completes the pharmacy order form. We've just finished checking the metronidazole and are onto midazolam when she puts the sheet down and sighs.

'Come on, Edie. Stop pretending you want to help with this bloody drugs check. Please talk. Stop holding everything in.'

'I don't know if I *can* tell you everything, Jaz.' She folds her arms tightly, in one of her moods where she won't take no for an answer. I relent. 'Okay then, but not now. I'll tell you more later. I'm meeting Harry after work; I'm going across to his department once everyone's out of the way. I'd actually like you to come with me, if you can?'

'Of course. Why though?'

'I don't mean to sound delicate, but just recently he has been a bit… I don't know. Just not himself. Angry. Particularly where his father is concerned.'

'Angry? Harry? No, I don't buy it.'

'I know, I know. To be honest, it's probably just me overreacting. But I think it would help if we all talked this through together. Plus, that bloody building of theirs gives me the creeps.'

'So meet him at the pub, then.'

'We don't want to be seen together. We're supposed to be separated.'

'Okay. But I'll have to leave by eight. I'm back on nights, I've taken an overtime shift.'

'Nights? Jaz, can't you cancel it?

'I need the money.'

I smile ruefully. 'Yeah, don't we all? Look, I'd better get back to theatres. Let's talk later. And thank you for being there.'

'I'm doing it because you're my mate. I'm looking out for you.'

In the empty corridor outside, I lean against the wall. Jaz was hinting I am paranoid, and not for the first time. What if it's the perfect word for me, for the way I'm acting? I have kept strong for so long; the thought of some kind of breakdown terrifies me. Claydon Manor terrifies me. The power and control they have over their patients terrifies me. Keep coping, keep coping. Keep going. Be strong. These words are now feeling emptier than ever.

Beyond where I'm standing, not more than twenty metres away, is the entrance to the main ICU. The department is empty; two of the bays' curtains are drawn. Matt's voice comes from behind one. *Ready, brace, roll.* The team must be turning a patient, which is a slow process. I've got a few minutes with no one around. I can make it to Cox's bay without being seen.

He might be sedated, but I know he can still hear me.

35

Samuel Cox

That Saturday morning, the abduction had been simpler than he thought. As he'd driven Edie away, heading towards the M11, no one had paid them a blind bit of notice. Jenny had left the house to go to the local shops, as she had done every Saturday. Michael – the man who he would have happily killed if he'd have been in the house at the time – was at golf. Edie was alone for half an hour. It was a warm spring day. Jenny hadn't even locked the door.

Is it the car engine he can hear in the background of his drifting thoughts, or just the hum of the ICU machines?

Her young voice carries to him.

'Where are we going, Sam?'

'I'm taking you back to the coast.'

'Will Sophie be there?'

'Not this time.'

'Just me and you?'

'Yeah.'

He had asked her questions as they drove, his morbid, unsatisfied curiosity getting the better of him.

'Do you love Michael, Edie?'

She hadn't answered, but in the rear-view mirror he could see her face crumple into a scowl, and could see her eyes glisten. And then he had known for sure that his suspicions were right. His chest had filled with bitter kind of relief, as the certainty spread that no matter what happened he had done the right thing.

'Edie. I don't want to upset you, but does he hurt you? Does he do bad things?'

Silence again. Was that a nod? The quietest whisper he had ever heard.

'Sometimes.'

He had lapsed into silence, unable to push any further, unwilling to keep tearing at an open wound. He thought his hatred for Jenny's husband couldn't get any deeper, any more all-consuming, but in Edie's broken expression was the proof that it could.

Afterwards – he doesn't remember how many days later – he had studied her face as he explained what was going to happen. People were going to come for them, and she must tell the truth when they did. It must come from her, because they wouldn't believe him if he told them himself.

'You see, taking you away was a bad thing, Edie.'

'No, it wasn't. I like being with you.'

'But for the people who come, it was a bad thing. They won't understand.'

As the net closed in, he had played with the idea of killing them both, rather than let her be taken away again. But he was a coward. He knew when the knock came, he couldn't do it. He wasn't even brave enough to kill himself, so he certainly couldn't kill her. Instead, he kept talking to her. Coaching her. Some men will come soon, Edie. I want you to tell them what your daddy did to you, okay? It's okay to tell them.

And he would tell them everything too; he would say why he had taken her away. They would not believe him, but he could try. Michael Carter was an influential man. He had powerful friends. But nothing would be more powerful than seeing the truth in this young girl's eyes. Maybe, if Edie could find a way to say what had happened to her, things would be okay.

When they had come for them, they had looked for the obvious solution, as he knew they would. They had looked for the easy target. And he knows now that he had asked too much of her. Edie hadn't been able to say it was Michael; she couldn't bring herself to tell them the name of the man who had been systematically abusing her. She was still too scared of him. When she admitted that these terrible things had happened to her, but refused to say who, it had been Sam they attached the guilt to. In the months and years afterwards he would torture himself, imagining her in the interview room. She was always shy, always scared of strangers. She would have said exactly what they wanted, and she would have kept her secrets to herself.

They gave him a choice. Those blank-faced men, the female officers who could hardly bear to look at him. Either he denies everything, and Edie is put through the trauma of a trial, or he saves her the horror of testifying and confesses. What terrible effects on her might a trial have? Their eyes hardened. Haven't you done enough already to hurt that young girl, Sam?

They worked on him for what felt like days, and he confessed. Through tears and groans of anguish, he told them what they wanted to hear, so he could save her. Except it didn't save her. In trying to spare her even more pain, he made it worse. He confessed to something he would rather have died than do to her, and they gave her back to Michael anyway. Jenny Carter stayed quiet too; she let him rot. She was as scared of Michael as Edie was. After everything, they gave her back to the man who had tormented her. Then he knew he had let her down, he had failed her.

And this is why he must be forgiven. That is why he had cut those words into his skin. *Edie Carter, forgive me.* He doesn't crave forgiveness for the abduction, for stealing her away from Michael and Jenny.

He needs forgiveness for delivering her back to them.

At first, he had managed to cling on to all the things that made taking her feel like the right thing to do. He remembers how she held him when he put her to bed that first night, grateful to be safe again, and he realised that, whatever the consequences, he had not just stood by and watched her suffer. He knew for certain that whatever happened afterwards, in that one moment, she knew that he loved her. So how had he let that certainty slip away? Over the years, why hadn't he clung onto that knowledge?

And what choice did he have but to keep living? To keep suffering.

To be tormented and hated, so that one day she would know how sorry he was for letting that monster have her back.

And there was more pain still to come. He was allowed newspapers in prison, and he could sometimes use the internet in the library. He had read about Sophie's disappearance on a local news summary. A brief report on the BBC Southwest news website, barely a paragraph. *Girl, 12, missing from Somerset care home. Coastguard search finds nothing.*

A small photograph, a short description of the search. By the next day, the news had moved on, as it always does. But for a moment he remembered that summer, the happiest of his life. Jenny was there, when they were still friends. Sophie. Edie. A makeshift family.

As his thoughts float, he can hear a quiet voice near him.

'Sam.'

Edie? Older, though No longer a child.

'I know what happened to you. It wasn't your fault.'

She is close to him again.

'I don't know if you can hear me, Sam. But I'm sorry for what you went through, I'm so sorry.'

She understands, finally.

'I'll make it better.'

Barely a whisper.

'I promise.'

36

Harry

I pretend to be hard at work writing up notes until everyone has left the department offices. The secure unit stays open all night, of course; its lights burn far into the night, but here everyone goes home between five and six. Wilson and I ignore each other now wherever possible; she avoids me studiously, just as careful of a conflict of interest as I am. We will never make close colleagues now, not that we ever were, and we exist in an uneasy, fragile truce. Along the corridor at five-ten, I hear her door close and the clack of her heels ticking along the battered parquet floor. She passes my office without slowing. She never stays past five-thirty any more, for obvious reasons. The others leave soon after, either waving as they pass, or calling in a quick goodbye. Then I am alone, pipes creaking and clicking as the ancient building exhales. I turn off my computer and fire a text off to Edie.

Everyone's left.

Okay. Be over soon.

She doesn't need to know about the letter from my father, which was waiting for me when I got home yesterday. I didn't expect him to take my angry comment literally, but as soon as I saw it lying on the mat in the hallway I knew it was from him. His slanted handwriting was a giveaway, as was the expensive stationery. Naturally, he was going to find a way of having the last word after I'd refused to take his calls. My mother has tried to play go-between since I told her Edie had moved out to Jaz's flat, but she soon gave up. I feel sorry for her because she's caught in the middle, between husband and son. In the kitchen I'd held the unread letter for several long moments, turning it in my hands. Then, I decided. Ripping it in half was difficult, but once the first tear was done I didn't stop. It was remarkably satisfying for such a petulant act. Soon, the letter was just paper fragments, floating down into in the bin. Screw him; as far as I'm concerned, it's too late for him and me to ever reconcile. But not too late for him to do what he can to ruin my relationship with Edie.

A noise in the corridor is a welcome diversion, but I'm surprised to hear two sets of footsteps approaching. Jaz follows Edie into my office and closes the door behind her. She is wearing a beanie hat, jeans and a baggy jumper, and she sits in one of my armchairs, crossing her legs.

She gazes around the room. 'God, what a gloomy office. I'm depressed just being here.'

I ignore her and frown at Edie. She reads the question in my eyes.

'I thought Jaz could tag along. She's part of this too.'

'Is she?' I shake my head. Edie's assumption that I wouldn't mind Jaz being here pisses me off. 'In what way, exactly?'

'Harry, Jaz and I talk all the time. She knows what's been going on. Anyway, I invited her.'

'Without checking with me first? Jesus.' I realise my voice is edging louder. The quick glance that Jaz flashes at Edie isn't lost on me, so I take some deep breaths. Nice and calm, Harry. 'Okay, whatever. Hello, Jaz.'

'Bad day, Doctor Creighton?'

'Yeah, something like that.' Her sarcasm is the last thing I need. I force a wry smile. 'Anyone want a coffee, now we're all here?'

Jaz nods. 'Seeing as I'm working and can't have anything stronger.'

I have several armchairs dotted around the room because of group sessions and, as I pass around the mugs, it feels like we're in group therapy. I don't know how I feel about us sharing everything like this together; I like Jaz and I know she and Edie are inseparable, but the news I want to tell Edie is not something Jaz is going to be able to help with. Jaz strikes me as someone who doesn't question authority in any serious respect. Perhaps on the surface she will make a show of defiance in certain situations, a stab at autonomy, but underneath she believes in hierarchy. Deep down, she thinks that the system is always right.

I glance between them. 'Okay, but can we talk openly, though?'

'Yes, Harry,' Edie insists. 'Jaz knows everything that we know.'

I keep my counsel and sip my coffee. She doesn't know everything we know, Edie, and if she did she wouldn't want anything to do with either of us. 'Right,' I now feel like I'm leading the session. 'So what exactly *do* we know?'

'That Sophie's dead,' Edie states bluntly.

'How do you know that?' I ask.

'Because I was there. The photo is dated two thousand and three. Sophie went missing in two thousand and eight. My mother kept taking me to the coast each year, for four years after the abduction. Four years after my father... died.'

'Wait a minute,' Jaz says. 'She's missing maybe, but you don't know she's dead.'

'I've seen her in flashbacks, Jaz. She drowned. It's the strongest, clearest memory I have. I spoke to the coastguard. It's an estuary; they said a body could be washed away and never found. I was the one who reported her missing that day.'

'There's something else that occurred to me about that photo.' They both turn to me as I speak. 'We still don't know how your mother and Samuel Cox were friends. Did your families know each other? We've been skirting around it for the last two weeks.'

'Yes, well it's a bit hard to find out when my mother was so traumatised by our visit that she decided to voluntarily put herself in an institution.'

The answer is obvious to me, but Edie can't or won't see it, and my suspicions are only going to make things worse if they're right. Her mother and Samuel Cox lived in the same area. They were friends. Okay, but what if they were more than that? When I look back, I sensed something in Jenny's eyes at the house, when Edie said he had come back into their lives. Before the hatred flared, before the barrier came back up, there was a moment of vulnerability. She was unguarded. The revulsion towards Samuel Cox now seems like a well-rehearsed act. Something she has convinced herself of over the years.

'Edie, why don't you spare you and your mother the pain?' Jaz leans forward, emphatic. 'I can see what it's doing to you. Why not forget Sophie? She's just a part of your life that doesn't exist any more. *Forget* Samuel Cox. The only thing that matters is getting yourself well today. Getting your head straight *right now*.'

'How could you say that to me? This is my life, *right now*.'

'I want the best for you, that's all.'

'Where have I heard that before?' Edie picks her thumb furiously.

'All right.' Jaz is briefly offended. 'It's not my business. I can tell I'm not wanted here.'

Edie glances at me, then stares at the ceiling and groans in frustration. 'I'm sorry, Jaz. I'm just… stressed.'

'Let's just call it a day,' I suggest. 'We're going around in circles. Edie, let's go for a drink.'

After a minute of thoughtful silence, Edie turns to me. 'No. Let's talk this through, Harry. Your father feels fine about investigating me, right?' With a sidelong look at Jaz, she continues, not waiting for an answer. 'So let's have a look at *him*.'

'What do you mean?'

'Let's work out why he's doing this, shall we?' She sits up in her chair. 'Let's see if we can find some skeletons in *his* closet.'

'There aren't any,' I tell her.

'How do you know he's so squeaky clean? He clearly doesn't mind overprescribing sedatives. So how do you know there's no dirt on him?'

'Because I've already looked.'

Earlier that afternoon, I'd drifted into the office of Beth Lafferty. We sat and talked about nothing for a while over the blisteringly strong coffee she made but we both knew I was there for advice. She stared at me as though she could see into my thoughts and asked the real reason I was there.

'How well do you know my father, Beth?' I replied.

'This sounds suspiciously like the opening of a therapy session, Harry.'

I laughed, but her curved, crow's feet eyes were mirthless. I knew immediately she was going to see through the bullshit I was about to give her, but I hoped she liked me well enough by now to indulge me.

'Yeah, I know. Don't worry, I don't have father issues,' I lied. 'His sixtieth birthday is coming up, and I've got a small speech to make. I've realised I don't know all that much about his career. I guess I avoided too much information, you know? Sometimes it's hard to measure up.'

'It depends what parameters you measure yourself by.' A wry smile played at the edge of her thin lips. 'Personally, I think you've got a different agenda to his, Harry. You're cut from different cloth.'

'I hope so.'

'And more honest?'

'Maybe.'

'So why don't you tell me the truth, instead of this sixtieth birthday bullshit?'

I smiled and nodded; naturally she'd seen through the lie. I admitted that my father was trying to split Edie and me up. How he was willing to do whatever it took to discredit her, and that we were pretending to go along with it until Edie qualified. So any ammunition she could give us against him would help.

Then, after smiling and thanking me for confiding in her, she talked as knowledgeably about my father as if she'd researched his life for a thesis. She knew where he had studied, because he had told her once at a conference, which he would have long forgotten. He went to the same college at Cambridge as me. Of course he did, the tutors there never stopped mentioning it. She told me where he had worked, his first jobs, what research positions he'd had. She told me what papers he'd published, and which journals he'd peer-reviewed. She knew which committees he'd sat on, the name of all the think tanks he'd contributed to over the years, even which mental health policies he'd advised on. She told me the year he'd got his professorship, even the name of the person he had taken over from at the Royal College. It was a potted biography from memory. I found out that, apart from being a shit father and a terrible husband, his cupboard is bare of bones. But there's something else, Harry, she said, and leaned forward conspiratorially.

Edie and Jaz are both waiting for me to expand my answer, so I precis what Beth Lafferty told me.

'My father is as clean as they come. He took the best-trodden path to the top of the tree you could imagine. A bit like the one he's put me on, before either of you say it.'

'Okay, why do I sense a but coming…?' Jaz asks.

'Because there is a but,' I reply. 'A big one. Beth Lafferty told me she overheard one of Amy Wilson's phone conversations. Beth was smoking outside, and Amy's window was open. You know how strident Amy's voice is.' I look at Edie. 'Edes, she was talking about us. She was telling whoever was on the phone that we were still together.'

'How does she know?'

'I don't know, but no prizes for guessing who she was probably talking to.' Edie looks at Jaz, wide-eyed. Jaz is shaking her head. 'He knows we've defied him, Edes,' I continue. 'And he's going to come for you. I don't know what he'll do next, but we have to be careful. If we're going to get to your exams, we'll have to be one step ahead of him.'

Edie is silent, pale.

'Edie, what are you thinking?' Jaz asks, concerned.

'That I need that drink,' she replies.

37

Samuel Cox

'What happens when you wake up? What will you say?'
      A voice drips into his consciousness. The past is clearer now; everything he sees is pure memory, a film running past his closed, taped-shut eyes. All of the nightmares have stayed away, but the outside world still intrudes in these random, fractured moments, which don't seem to matter so much any more.

The voice is different to Edie's but, in this clouded twilight world, everything seems to be her. It all blends into one. He talks to her in the darkness. What will I say when I wake up?

I'll tell you everything. They didn't believe me then, but maybe people will believe me now. If you can tell the truth as well, maybe they will believe us, and we can be together again?

And Jenny. Will she ever be whole again as well? Will she ever be able to rid herself of the guilt? What happened to her?

The gentle beeps of the monitor punctuate his drifting thoughts. Was the conversation real? He can't tell. Time doesn't matter any more. Years might have passed while he has been lying here.

He hears a different beeping, higher, more jarring. The pump. He recognises the pumps; he knows enough to understand how they are keeping him sedated. Someone is starting a new infusion.

Warmth begins to spread through his body. The warmth of the summer sun again, but different this time, more potent. A chemical warmth. But just as comforting, just as beautiful.

His thoughts begin to fade into darkness.

He has been getting better. He's heard them say so.

He will wake up and everything will be right again. Soon, he will wake up.

Edie, I will see you again.

Wake up.

38
Edie

Wake up.

Something pulls me from a dream, leaving me with an afterimage of a dark grey, swollen sea. I stare into the darkness, unable to go back to sleep, listening to the sounds of the night. Outside, a dog barks somewhere in the distance, the electric whine of a milk cart hums past the window. The bed is empty next to me. Harry is not here. We had gone for drinks after Jaz went to work; there was no point pretending we're separated any more. He'd asked if he could come back to her flat with me, and my instincts were warmly numb, fearless. Once we'd arrived back here, we'd shared a couple more drinks, talked, and gone to bed as if proving to ourselves it would take more than his father to tear us apart. The darkness still has that middle-of-the-night feel, and it's as if he were never here. I vaguely remember his phone ringing in the very small hours, him swearing softly under his breath. He'd got out of bed and left; there was an emergency in the secure unit.

Wake up, I tell myself. Get up. There is no point in lying here. The images it brings are too troubling, the feelings too dark and suffocating. I look at my phone, mildly hungover. 3.30 a.m. My thoughts drift to the ICU. No matter what else I try to think of, it always comes back to Samuel. Jaz's flat is in Edgbaston, twenty minutes away from the hospital. I'm not on shift until eight, but I'm not sure I could bear pacing around the flat for another four hours. I pull myself from the bed and quickly shower, letting the water run cool for a while to blast the last of the night's sleep away.

Morris is not on nights this week; he won't be in the department for several hours. I throw my work bag over my shoulder and leave the flat. Outside, the early June morning is cool, with a line of denim blue beyond the houses, a shade lighter than the cobalt colour of the night. Stars are still dotted white across the sky, but the beginning of day is pushing them gradually back towards the western horizon. In the car, the early morning DJ is annoyingly bright and cheerful, so I turn the radio off, driving through the quiet streets with only my thoughts for company, and the nagging sense of unease that pulled me from sleep.

Apart from the Emergency Department, which is never completely quiet, the hospital corridors are empty as I walk towards ICU. I did a stint on the retrievals team when I was doing my surgical placement; those grim visits to harvest organs from other hospitals always seemed to happen at night. The epitome of night work. Ever since then, I've associated the silence of hospital corridors at night with that kind of secrecy. But as I turn the corner towards theatres and ICU, the sound of running plastic soles hitting the vinyl floor reaches my ears. It grows louder, and I turn to see a figure in blue scrubs fly past me. I recognise Dylan, the night ODP from theatres, bleep in hand, his lanyard swinging and bouncing as he runs. Running like this at night can only mean one thing: he's answering an arrest call. I speed up, following him through the doors of ICU and into the main department. Stark against the muted lighting of the department, the overhead lights are bright in one bay. My heart leaps into my throat. Bay Four.

Something has happened to Samuel Cox.

When I get to the bed, Jaz is kneeling on it, directly over Cox, her hands locked together, arms rigid, her fist planted in the middle of his exposed chest, pumping up and down. With every chest compression she does, she and Cox bounce and sink into the mattress. In one sick, head-swimming moment, I realise he is in cardiac arrest. I register details with a heightened, adrenaline-fuelled awareness. From the fading scars on his chest where Jaz's gloved hands are, to the compression waveforms on the monitor. Dylan is busy checking the endotracheal tube and pulling the drawers of the resuscitation trolley open.

As I run to the bedside, Jaz stares at me, disbelief and confusion in her eyes.

'Edie? What the fuck?'

'Jaz, what's happened?'

Her words come in staccato bursts as she exerts herself with the compressions.

'Sudden… deterioration. Ventricular… arrhythmias. Then into… cardiac arrest.'

'Who's the consultant on call?'

'Jeremy Dacre.'

'He's held up in the ED,' Dylan says, hitting the CPR button on the bed. The air mattress deflates, and he takes over compressions from Jaz. Dylan is heavy set and muscular; the compression waveforms on the ECG are already increasing.

'Okay, I'll lead,' I tell them. For now, Cox has ceased to exist as a person; he is a patient in need of resuscitation and I have no past with him, no connection or relationship. Nothing else exists except the cardiac arrest. 'Let's see what rhythm we have.'

Dylan pauses CPR and we all turn to the screen, scanning the ECG trace. It's a series of jagged, irregular peaks and troughs. Ventricular fibrillation.

'Okay, VF. Back on compressions.'

As Dylan continues pushing, I rush to the defibrillator and pull the pads from it, peeling off the packaging. Working around Dylan's muscular, tattooed arms, I attach the sticky pads to Cox's scarred chest.

'Get some adrenaline ready, Jaz.' I try to keep my voice quiet, steady. As a foundation year doctor I was always told the noisier the resuscitation, the worse it was being run. As Jaz dips into the resus trolley, another nurse appears, her blonde ponytail bobbing as she runs to the bed. Heather, newly qualified. I've only worked with her a couple of times. I hope she's a quick learner.

'Okay, stop CPR, Dylan.' I check the screen. More jagged lines. As Dylan starts compressions again I charge the defibrillator, hearing the whine, listening to the high-low alert when the shock is ready to be delivered.

'VF. Stand clear.' My voice carries in the silent unit. Dylan steps away.

'Clear,' he calls.

My eyes scan the bed. The flashing button on the defibrillator hums under my fingertips.

'Shocking *now*.' I press the button and the defibrillator, full of potential energy like a large dog straining at a leash, sends two hundred joules into Cox's chest. His upper body lifts from the bed in an exaggerated shrug.

'Back on the chest, please, Dylan. Alternate with Heather every two minutes. Jaz, first adrenaline please.'

Jaz hands me the prefilled syringe, and I push it into a spare port on Cox's central line, calling the time. There are two minutes in the cycle before the next shock, enough time to think ahead. I turn to Jaz.

'Reversible causes, Jaz. Any ideas?'

'No, I don't know.'

'Come on, you were here. What happened?'

'Nothing.' Jaz is fraught. 'Jesus, Edie. He just arrested, that's all.'

'Right, let's get some urgent bloods done. I want everything, urea and electrolytes, blood sugar, troponin. Come on, think. Something must have caused this.'

Jaz shakes her head, *I don't know*, then starts to draw blood. I run through possible causes. Airway? I rush to the head of the bed, but the tube looks fine. The capnograph on the monitor shows the ventilator is doing its job.

'Two minutes is up,' Jaz says, her voice cracking. She is normally calmer than this.

'Okay, stop CPR, Dylan.' I glance at the screen. 'VF. Stand clear.'

'Clear.'

Another pause, then my finger finds the shock button again. 'Shocking *now*.'

The energy leaps through him and Cox's torso lifts again, his arms jumping. We all glance at the screen. Still VF.

'Dylan, run that blood, please. Heather, take over compressions. Where is Doctor Dacre?' I quietly go through all of the reversible causes for cardiac arrest. If I can work out what caused it, I stand a better chance of keeping him alive. As the resuscitation continues, I listen to his chest. It sounds fine, no pneumothorax. What then? Toxicity? Low oxygen? No, not in here, surely. 'Jaz, was his saturation okay prior to this?'

She glances up from the resuscitation trolley. 'It was fine. He just went into a series of arrhythmias.'

'Okay. When can we expect those electrolytes?'

'They'll take a few minutes,' Heather calls from the bed, where she is performing perfect nursing-school compressions. She looks incredibly young as she kneels by Cox's side, her wilted ponytail falling down across the side of her face.

'What's happening?' A voice behind me pulls my attention away from the resuscitation. Instead of Jeremy Dacre coming around the corner, I see a tall figure, approaching in a fast, controlled step I recognise all too well. Richard Morris pushes his glasses back on his nose. 'Edie, what are you doing here? You're not on nights.'

'Neither are you.' This isn't the time for a row, but my hackles are raised.

'I'm second on-call. We'll deal with this later.' He looks at the resuscitation unfolding in front of him. 'Right, fill me in.'

I take a breath, pushing the unanswered questions away. 'Jaz reported sudden unidentified arrhythmias, then VF arrest. I arrived with CPR in progress. Two shocks so far, still VF. Bloods requested.'

'Any ideas of cause yet?'

'Either metabolic or a toxicity of unknown origin.'

'Okay. Jaz, relieve Heather please. Heather, could you get another adrenaline and some amiodarone ready, please. Is it time for the third shock yet?'

As Morris takes over and the situation finally sinks in, I get an intense, almost serene, sense of time stopping. I take in every detail of the scene before me. Samuel Cox seems older than ever before. No longer the young man on the beach. Not even the man in prison, carrying his past and his guilt, and being reminded of it with every punch and act of violence or stream of verbal abuse. Just an old man.

A body. A patient hovering between life and death. The scars on his chest are vivid against his pale skin. The words he had cut into himself.

Edie Carter. Forgive me.

I can see the glances of the resuscitation team. I can sense the energy slipping away from them as the resuscitation drags on and nothing improves.

I can feel the hope fading.

39

Edie

The bay is quiet now, the aftermath of the resuscitation is everywhere. Morris called time on it fifteen minutes ago. *Time of death*, he announced, *four thirty-six*.

I know we could have done more. We could have tried for longer. But we didn't.

I'd let Morris know how I felt, telling him he'd called it too soon, and he'd stormed off to the desk to write his notes. Jaz is at the desk too, preparing for the final drugs round. Life in ICU goes on. She is pale, shocked; it's obvious she is struggling to concentrate. Wearily, I begin tidying. The defibrillator pads now lie on the floor; empty syringes of adrenaline and amiodarone litter the top of the trolley; fluid bags, giving sets and monitor leads lie jumbled across the bed. I pull the curtains across for privacy. It's not my job to tidy up the bay, but I can't stand to see him lying in all the mess. Apart from telling Morris how I felt about ending the resuscitation, I haven't raged or cried, or shown any emotion. But the emotion is all there, buried deep.

Cox is still and pale, and the marks on his chest that are visible above the loose-fitting neck of the hospital gown seem to have faded into his skin, as if he has absorbed them in death. He doesn't look young again; it's a myth that years of care fall off people when they die. But he does look tranquil. The machines are quiet; the ventilator is off, the monitor is a blank, dark screen. I want to deflate the cuff on his endotracheal tube and slide it out of his mouth, remove the central intravenous line from his neck, dabbing any dark post-mortem bleeding pearling the skin with a cotton swab. I want to remove all the dressings and drains, which make him look like a patient, to somehow make him whole again. But there will almost certainly be an autopsy, and I don't want to give Morris anything else to criticise me for, so I leave them in place. Instead, I gently make sure the dead man's eyes are fully closed, then pull the collar of his gown higher. I wipe the corners of his mouth and remove all the medical debris I can from the arrest. I take down the metronidazole, detach the pumps, the fluids. Everything goes in the clinical waste, as I do what I can to make Samuel Cox look less of a victim.

I study his face. There is no sorrow in me, just numbness. When I do start processing what happened, there will be regret. Anger, maybe. A deep sense of injustice. I lift his lids for the last time, but there is nothing there any more. I once knew a junior doctor who would look into the eyes of the deceased as if to see where the soul had gone. She came from a religious family and was wrestling with her own faith, her belief that there is a plan for the cosmos. I can understand that now, but it takes superhuman faith to believe there is any logic to such a lottery.

What impulse was it that woke me up in the darkness two hours ago, that kept me from sleeping? What force got me out of bed to come here at precisely this time? I don't believe in a sixth sense, but I do believe that true accidents are rare. Like Morris being here, for example.

Talk of the devil. The curtains swish open and his gaunt face pokes around them. 'Doctor Carter? I think we need to speak.'

It is now five o'clock, and the hospital is coming to life. The morning cleaners are arriving, and some deliveries are being made to the cafeteria and the kitchen. The bleeps of reversing lorries making deliveries are outside, the clatter of storage cages being pushed echoes along corridors. Upstairs, the offices are quiet, but Morris's door is unlocked. I follow him inside, and he perches on a corner of the desk. I decide to stand, despite feeling weary to my bones.

'Well?' he says. 'Why do I find you at this resuscitation when I arrive?'

'I came in early because I couldn't sleep. When I realised a resuscitation was in progress on the unit, I helped. Despite our agreement, not to have attended would have been negligent.' He sighs and rubs his chin. He knows I'm right. I may have made mistakes in the past, but this is one thing he can't hold against me. 'And why were *you* in so early this morning, Doctor Morris?'

'Not that I have to explain myself to you, but I am second on-call and Doctor Dacre knew he was going to be in the ED for the next few hours. So I came in from home when Doctor Dacre called for backup, in case anything else happened. It was a good job I did.'

A glance around the room tells me the couch along the back wall of Morris's office has been used. The cushions are indented, and I can see where a hospital blanket has been hurriedly tossed under the couch. He didn't come in from home; he was here all night. I can't help but think of him and Wilson, and I pity his family, grinning obliviously from the photo on his desk. On-call duties are a perfect cover for an affair.

'More to the point,' he continues, 'I want to discuss your attitude during the resuscitation.'

'What do you mean?'

He walks around the desk and sits, motioning for me to take a seat. I remain standing and he lets it go with a brief snort. 'I mean your lack of professionalism. I am the consultant; when I call the end of the resuscitation, you comply, Doctor Carter. You do not try to continue.'

'You asked if everyone was in agreement. I was not, and I made that clear.'

'You couldn't give a valid reason why we should continue. We had exhausted all possibilities. Until we have an autopsy, we cannot possibly know what caused it.'

'It was an in-hospital arrest; we could have gone on for longer, done more tests.'

'Enough, Doctor Carter.' He stands again, comes around the desk and stands before me. 'I want you to go home today, Doctor Drake can do the general list on his own. There are a couple of FY1 doctors who need some experience too. They can assist him. Go home. You're supernumerary today.'

'You can't get rid of me again.'

'I'm not getting rid of you; I'm giving you today off. Take it.'

I walk to the door, but something makes me stop and turn. 'We could have saved him. You could have woken him up ten days ago; he was improving. Were you scared of what he might say or something?'

Morris's face contorts in a sneer. 'Scared? Watch your step, doctor.'

'Yes, scared. Both you and James Creighton.'

'What are you suggesting?' He comes closer; beneath the simmering anger there is a pointed threat. His voice is quiet but intense, and he has crossed the threshold of my personal space. The room instantly becomes uncomfortable, menacing. I'm on a floor of the hospital with nobody on it except Richard Morris and myself, so I back towards the door, and put my hand on the handle. He doesn't move with me, and the space between us makes me breathe a little easier. I could tell him about Creighton and his manipulation. His unethical collaboration with Amy Wilson. The affair. I could blow the lid on everything right now if I wanted. Yes, including my career. I rein my anger in.

'All I'm suggesting is he could have been woken up.'

'Once again, you're overstepping the mark. Be careful.' His intense stare remains. 'I'll be launching an investigation into the arrest this morning. There will be an autopsy within the next forty-eight hours.'

'Will you be pushing it through quickly then?'

'Yes, of course.'

'Good.' I fix my gaze on him, watching his reaction to what I am about to say. 'Because for your information, Cox wasn't guilty of anything except trying to protect me. Do you realise that? He may have abducted me, but he didn't abuse me.'

'Let me tell you something, Edie. You're coming across as very unpredictable. Erratic. You know, I told Doctor Wilson this might happen if we took you back too soon.' He leans into my space again. There is intensity in his gaze, but his voice is level. 'I questioned whether you were ready.'

'Stop pretending. You're in Wilson's pocket. At the very least you could admit you're glad Cox is dead. '

He points towards the door. 'Go home, Edie, and think carefully about how many of these accusations you want to make public.' His eyes are cold. 'It's the weekend tomorrow. Come back on Monday with your emotions under control, and I will forget what I heard here this morning.'

I leave with one last look at Morris, his stare fixed on me. Then, finally, the delayed reaction begins. As I make my way through the corridors and out past the Emergency Department entrance. Two ambulances are there, the crews cleaning the back, watching me with curiosity as I stumble past. The morning is now a pale blue-yellow, and the eastern part of the sky is a long white strip of cloud. I stare upwards, the blue blurring and flickering as the tears begin. I fumble in my bag for my phone.

I know it's early, Harry, but pick up. Please pick up.

'Edie?' he mumbles.

'Where were you?'

'Edes, I've just got back into bed. One of our patients attempted suicide on the unit in the early hours, they called me in. What's the matter?'

The words catch in my throat, but I manage to get them out. 'Samuel Cox is dead.'

His voice is thick with sleep. 'What?'

'He's dead, Harry. This morning.'

'How?'

'I don't know yet. But I rang to say I'm having it out with your father, once and for all.'

Immediately, he is awake, his voice alert. 'No, Edie. You're upset. Tired. Don't do anything now. Come home.'

'No, Harry. I've had it, I'm going over there.'

'Please, Edie. I'm begging you. Don't confront him.' I can hear his breathing, hard and fast. He is close to panic. 'It's what he wants. Trust me.'

'What do I do then?' I am sobbing now. I don't care that the paramedics are watching me. 'This has to end now. What do I do?'

219

'We wait for the right time, Edie. In a few months you're qualified. You're free. We can make it that far. Come home to *our* house. Let's be together. Talk.'

'And what about your father?'

Harry's breathing is calmer now; he recognises that I'm wavering. My moment of irrational rage has passed. In his voice, panic gives way to determination.

'My father? Leave him to me.'

40

Edie

Harry and I have spent the weekend holed up in the house. If Creighton already knows we're still together, we may as well stop pretending. Where James Creighton is concerned, I can't stick my head in the sand forever, but ignoring the situation for a few days has felt good. It has been like old times, where me and Harry used to end up in pyjamas at seven in the evening and watch back-to-back films surrounded by takeaway pizza. Switching my thoughts off is a form of protection; it's me saying I don't want to tackle whatever comes next. At least not for a while. Harry has been kind and attentive, like he used to be. No flashes of anger, resentment or frustration. It is as if something in his mind has clarified, some cloud has dispersed, and positivity has settled in its place. Like me, he hasn't wanted to talk about the situation, but it's as though a plan has formed in his mind, and he sees a way forward. For me, everything is static; after my impulse to confront Harry's father the morning Samuel Cox died, all the energy evaporated. Cox is dead, now only the problem of James Creighton remains, and I don't want to face it yet.

My only contact with work has been to ring Jaz to tell her I'm back at home. We spoke for an hour on Friday afternoon when she'd woken up following her night shift, but the conversation was stilted. Nights do horrible things to your energy anyway, even without an unsuccessful resuscitation. She already looked frazzled by the time Morris called me up to his office after the arrest, so I knew she would crash out as soon as she got back to the flat. But even with the post-nights slump, she sounded beaten.

'Morris won't even talk to me, Edie,' she murmured. 'It's like I've committed some kind of crime, just by being the one who found Cox in arrest.'

She sounded more downbeat than I'd ever heard her before. She'd had depression in the past, peaks and troughs, but nothing like this. I tried to pick her up, even though my positivity was drained too. 'You're a great nurse Jaz, Morris is a dick.' But none of it worked. Nothing of her effervescence remained. Even with me, her best friend, she sounded resentful, as if I was part of some conspiracy against her. A barrier had come down.

Now I'm stretched out on the sofa, my laptop propped on my stomach, in the same position I've been in for most of the weekend. The usual Sunday evening programmes are on television, but I'm not taking any notice, and Harry is in the kitchen making cheese on toast. Healthy living hasn't topped our priorities this weekend, and we're in a place where nothing matters outside of the two of us and our work. I'll keep my head down. I'll have polite chats with Morris and Wilson, attend sessions. There is nothing now to prevent me being allowed back into ICU. Unless Creighton carries through on his threats, which I'm desperately hoping were empty, Morris will sign more of my competencies, and I'll qualify. Completing my training is now my only concern. It's incredible how you can switch certain parts of your mind off, at least temporarily, taking each day as it comes, convincing yourself that ignorance is bliss.

I hit a couple of buttons on the keyboard and refresh my emails. While Harry and I might have been physically inert, lacking the emotional energy and willpower to do anything other than exist together, I've at least tried to get closure on certain things. Another email pops into my inbox, part of a chain that has been bouncing back between me and Claydon Manor for the past couple of days. This one, sent an hour ago, has a tone of finality. Anyone checking emails on a Sunday afternoon means business. It is from Sue Willard, confirming that my mother is being held under a Section Three. I scan the email.

Your mother will be required to remain with us under observation for a period of six months, or until assessed fit by her clinician, whichever is the sooner... we do not see any conflict of interest in Professor Creighton's involvement in your mother's care, as you and he are not related... Please bear in mind that visits to your mother should now be arranged twenty-four hours in advance, although we will do our best to facilitate urgent visits.

Creighton had moved quicker than I could; he had already medicated her, and now he can keep her exactly where he wants her. He can talk to her, get whatever he wants out of her. But whatever he discovers needs to be proven. Michael was cremated, so there is no physical evidence of her giving the overdose, and the confession of a medicated woman means nothing. I'm more scared of him proving *my* mental health fragile. I am so drained I haven't even had the strength to fight my corner properly. Some angry emails and phone calls to the centre are all I've managed this weekend. I toyed with visiting, but had to make do with a slurring, medicated voice at the end of the phone.

Keep quiet if Creighton visits you, Mum, is all I could manage, even though it's too late, and she's already told him what she did. *You don't have to speak to him.*

The six o'clock news comes on; death, destruction, misery. I turn it off, shut the laptop and close my eyes, letting myself drift. I've been consumed with thoughts of the autopsy and what the pathologist might have found. At least I've been able to talk it over with Harry. I've run through everything that might have caused it no matter how unlikely; thrombus, toxic shock from the liver abscess, anaphylaxis, even intra-abdominal haemorrhage. It's all speculation.

On the coffee table, my phone buzzes. *Jaz.* I glance at the time; ten past six. She will be getting ready to go back on nights. Worried she might think I've been avoiding her, I reach across and swipe to answer. I hit the speaker option, and flop back on the sofa.

'Hey Jaz. I'm sorry I've been a bit absent this weekend. I've been sticking my head in the sand.'

'Edie, I'm through at the KG.' She sounds drunk. 'What the fuck have they done to me?'

'Jaz. Slow down. I don't understand.'

'I've been suspended,' she cries. 'They're saying I killed Samuel Cox.'

By seven, I'm knocking on her door. She opens it and I immediately take her in my arms. Her eyes are bloodshot, drying tears streaking her cheek. Her hair is down, hanging loosely except where it's plastered to the side of her face where she's been crying. She is in jeans and a hoodie, her work scrubs thrown in a pile on the floor. She pushes free of me, but I persuade her to sit on the sofa with me.

'Jaz, I don't know what they think happened, or why they're blaming you. But it can't be true.' I look at the coffee table; there is a bottle of brandy, half-empty. At this point, another drink isn't going to hurt her. I get another glass and pour some out for both of us. 'Can I get you anything?'

'No.' She looks like she is cried out, her eyes are wet, but she is no longer sobbing.

I wrap my arm around her shoulder. 'What have they been saying?'

I was wrong; she isn't cried out. The question sets her off again, and she drops her face into her hands, shaking her head. She tries to control her breathing and looks at me helplessly.

I wait, rubbing her back.

'Samuel Cox's autopsy,' she finally manages.

'Yes, what about it?'

'Cardiac toxicity,' she whispers. 'Opioid-induced cardiac toxicity. They say I caused it.'

'Wait a minute.' My mind is racing. 'You told me Morris prescribed morphine for the liver abscess. So how could they blame that on you?'

'Drug error.' Her sobs begin again, rising and falling, eventually petering out. 'They're saying I gave fentanyl instead of morphine. They're investigating me for negligence.'

'Shit, Jaz.' There is nothing I can say to her to make this better. Fentanyl is nearly one hundred times stronger than morphine, and in theatres and ICU they have buckets of it. The ampoules they use on theatre lists are jokingly called party-size; five hundred micrograms in ten millilitres. Enough to kill several times over. But the ampoules are completely different; there is no way they could be mistaken for morphine, not even on the arse end of a busy night shift.

'How could that happen? It's a controlled drug. Wasn't it double-checked when you drew it up?'

She nods. 'Of course. I got Matt to do it.'

'So you can't both be wrong.'

'I didn't ask him to sign though. I forgot. I could have sworn I had, but, when they checked, there was no signature. He's trying to take the blame himself, and they've taken his statement. But they said I gave it, so I'm culpable. It was nights, I was tired, but I didn't give fentanyl, I just know it.' The sobbing starts again, racking her body. 'Oh God, what's going to happen to me, Edie?'

Opioid overdose. Toxicity would have occurred within minutes. 'I wonder if they've done the autopsy quickly so they can release the body for cremation.'

She shrugs. 'Maybe. I don't know. That's the last thing I care about. Edie, if I lose my job I can't even… what are my family going to think?'

'Don't even go there, okay?'

'No, but what *will* people think? I couldn't bear it if they…' Her voice hitches, on the edge of hysteria. 'The job is everything to me, you know that.'

'Jaz, calm down. Breathe,' I say, making sure she meets my gaze. 'Think hard about what happened on Thursday night. Think about everything that led up to it, from the moment Samuel Cox arrived in our ICU. Write everything down all the events you can remember, everything you can think of that Morris said or did. Will you do that for me?'

She drops her face into her hands, her voice muffled. 'Yeah. But it won't help now, will it?'

'It might. It'll help us work out exactly how this happened. A fentanyl overdose would have been almost instant, Jaz. You didn't give it, so it must have been someone else in the hospital that night.

Morris was lying about coming in from home; he'd slept in his office. He was there all night. Write down everything you think is relevant, no matter how small.'

She stares at me. 'And what then?'

'We work out how this happened. Look, I know I sound paranoid, but just do it for me. Please. Think back over the last few weeks and write down every conversation, every thought, every detail. Then we can go through it together, see what you remember.'

'Edie, what are you trying to prove?'

'You might not have killed Samuel Cox, Jaz.' Her red-rimmed eyes are locked on mine. 'But someone did.'

41
Edie

There are no long, black limousines idling, no mourners gathered, no extravagant flower displays. The Sandwell Valley Crematorium car park is almost empty, and the waiting area near the red-brick arches of the entrance door is deserted. As Harry and I follow the grey tarmac path to the squat, newly built chapel, the only people we can see are the straggling mourners from the previous ceremony, reading messages in the covered brick cloister. No one is waiting to mourn Samuel Cox. We pass beyond the arches of the door, shaped like a hacienda-style ranch house, into the cool, clinical white and wood hall of the chapel. I was wrong about there being no other mourners; one person got here ahead of us and is sitting near the front. Harry and I have trebled the size of the congregation.

A slow, mournful string quartet piece, probably on loop, spills out of tinny speakers. Near the front, beyond the sea of empty seats, stands the hospital chaplain. This is a public service funeral, a hospital send-off for those with no relatives willing to foot the bill, and to say it is a no-frills affair would be generous. Samuel Cox's coffin, a bare, polished wooden casket, rests on the dais in front of the curtains it will disappear behind after the chaplain has mumbled a few words. I glance at Harry, not sure where to sit. Somewhere in the middle seems appropriate. The man at the front is in his late fifties, dressed the way men of certain means do when they are trying to make an effort. His dark-blue suit is cheap, but neatly pressed and clean, his iron-grey hair parted to the side, his black glasses framed in a severe horn-rim. On his lap, his hands fold across a dark, checked flat cap.

Harry takes my hand as we wait. He probably assumes I'll be emotional, but I've been strangely ready for this all week. I've been more concerned about Jaz. She has been monosyllabic since we saw each other, and sometimes won't take my calls at all. When I do get through to her, she is off the phone within a minute, making some excuse why she can't talk. So I'm not thinking of the service as much as trying to work out what I'll say to her when I visit her tomorrow. I've decided to go over and see her, to knock until she speaks to me. She has become withdrawn and isolated, and, after what they have done to her, it's a red flag that makes me very nervous.

The chaplain coughs to get our attention, the noise echoing. The empty chapel is beyond depressing. A single bouquet rests against the side of the dais and, seeming to notice it for the first time, the chaplain picks the flowers up and rests them on the coffin. He coughs again and looks at each of us in turn as if wondering whether it's worth the effort.

'We are gathered here to lay to rest the mortal remains of Samuel Cox,' he enunciates. 'Lord, may you forgive this man his sins and welcome his soul into your kingdom…'

His voice is sonorous, rising and falling in a devout singsong, as he repeats words he must have used a thousand times before. He drones on, talking about a man of which he knew nothing, hinting that, although we are all sinners, we're all redeemable should we repent. He doesn't touch upon whether he believed Samuel Cox had repented, remaining blissfully unaware that he didn't need to. He had nothing to atone for, there is nothing to be forgiven. After five minutes, the chaplain ends his address abruptly, as if realising he's exceeded his allotted time.

The curtains close and, with a brief smile at the tiny congregation, he tidies up his papers, and walks as quickly as dignity will allow from the dais. It's over, Samuel Cox is gone. Melanie didn't come; why would I have expected her to? The solitary mourner stands and walks to the front, and bows briefly to the cross on the front of the podium. As he turns, my pulse quickens. They look so similar, it's as if Samuel Cox has risen from the dead. The man makes his way down the aisle towards the entrance. Breathing faster, I let go of Harry's hand and follow. Outside, the man stops, sensing I'm behind him.

Closer, the likeness is even more uncanny. 'Sir, I'm sorry to bother you. I'm Doctor Carter. I helped look after Mr Cox for a short while.'

'I see. Thank you, Doctor Carter.' My surname hasn't registered with him; why would it? He extends his hand. 'Trevor Cox. I am… I *was*… Samuel's brother.' The moment hangs, then he sighs. 'I didn't think anyone else would be here. As a doctor, it's nice of you not to judge him. Very few people really knew him.'

'I think I knew him quite well.'

'Well, thank you for your care, miss. Everyone deserves some mourners, no matter what they've done.'

He fits his cap and turns to go.

'Sir, my full name is Edie Carter. I'm…' It's now or never. 'I was the girl your brother took.'

Under other circumstances, the confusion that contorts his features might look comical. He frowns at Harry, who meets his stare with a brief nod. A subtle, blink-and-you'll-miss-it confirmation of who I am.

'Why would you come here?' Trevor Cox manages eventually. His eyes are harder now, tempered with an unbearable look of guilt. 'Is it to dance on his grave?'

'No, not at all.'

'What he did wrecked the whole family, Miss Carter. I don't know what to say to you. How did you come to be looking after him? How could you bring yourself to do that?'

'Mr Cox, when he was released, your brother came to find me. He wanted to say sorry. He was… troubled.'

He removes his glasses and wipes his eyes. How do I tell him what really happened? How do I explain his brother was a good man? Trevor Cox glances at Harry as if he is looking for help.

'This is Harry, my fiancé,' I explain.

'Mr Cox, can we buy you a drink?' Harry asks.

*

The Royal Oak is a small corner pub on its last legs, with one late-morning drinker sitting at the end of the bar. We sit around an old-fashioned hammered brass table in the corner. The sunlight streams in, catching clouds of dust motes.

'I was always told we looked alike,' Trevor Cox is saying. He sips a dark-brown pint of something cloudy. 'But actually, I'm older by three years.'

'Were you still close after…?' Harry begins. His cheeks flush. 'I'm sorry,' he mumbles, 'that was clumsy.'

For the first time since we met a small, sad smile forms on Trevor's face. 'No, we weren't. In fact, we'd lost touch for a while before…' he glances at me, 'before it happened.' He trails off. 'We were close as kids. But how could you forgive something like that? Even your own brother?'

I'm torn. Could I change his mind about his brother in the five minutes we have? If we stayed for an hour, could I wipe out twenty years of guilt? Would it even matter? One day, I promise myself, I'll track Trevor Cox down again and tell him the real story. Today, the best I can manage is a shrug.

'I understand how you feel, Mr Cox. My job is to treat everybody the same, no matter what they've done.'

He gazes out of the window as if looking for an explanation in the clear late-spring sky. 'Well, thank you for what you did for my brother, doctor. And I'm sorry for what happened. For a long time on the drive here I questioned why I was coming. But he was the only blood relative I had left, and I know it was the right thing to do. You can't rationalise it any further than that really, can you?'

Something he said nags at me. 'No other blood relatives?'

'Well, I meant first-degree. I have a niece, but we don't see each other that often.' He swallows some of his pint.

'Sorry, Trevor.' Harry plants his elbows on the table. 'But do you have any other brothers or sisters?'

'No. My niece is Sam's daughter.'

'Yes, but she is dead, isn't she?' I can hear the doubt in my voice. 'I've spoken to Samuel's wife Melanie in the course of treating him, and she said their daughter was dead.'

Trevor laughs bitterly, then realises I am being serious. 'Dead? No, she's not dead. At least I hope not; I got a Christmas card from her last year. I knew she wouldn't come today; she hated her father more than her mother did, if that's possible.'

'But why would Melanie say their daughter was dead?'

He sighs. 'Melanie has distanced herself from everything to do with Samuel. She and her daughter had issues after what happened.' He pauses. 'Melanie couldn't cope. Their daughter went into care.'

Care? Harry's eyes are on me, but I can't look at him. 'What's her name?' My question is too abrupt, my voice too shrill.

'Lisa. She is Lisa Saunders now.'

My heart is pounding so hard it must be visible through my dark funeral jacket. Pain shoots through my thumb as my nail tears into the skin. 'Did she ever have any other names? Nicknames? Anything like that?'

He shakes his head. 'No, not that I remember.'

I reach in my bag and find a pen and scrap of paper. I suck the fresh blood from my thumb, aware of Harry's worried frown. 'Trevor, could you let me have her details, if you don't mind?'

'I don't know.'

'Please.'

There must be something in my tone, some deep urgency. He holds my eyes, then picks up the pen and begins writing. 'I suppose so. Why though?'

'It's a form of closure for me. I'd like to give her my condolences.'

Underneath the table, Harry has found my hand and is holding it as if to stop it shaking.

42

Harry

Outside in the car, Edie's sombre, dark-grey funeral suit feels out of place with her agitation. She's expecting me to play along with a theory I'm certain is wrong. 'What if she's changed her name, Harry? What if my flashback isn't what I think, and she's not dead? It's got to be her, right? How can you be so calm?'

'Because I think you're clutching at straws.'

'That's why we couldn't find any record of her in the registers or anything. There was no death certificate, no body turned up on the coastal search. She never drowned. That image I have of her struggling in the sea is just some twisted memory. She's changed her name.'

'Come on, Edie.' I start the car, turn the radio down and let the engine idle. 'It's a long shot, isn't it?'

'Just humour me for a moment, okay?'

'Okay. Go on then.' I lean on the steering wheel, allowing myself a wry smile. Edie wears her heart on her sleeve far more than she would ever admit, and sometimes her thought processes can be blindingly obvious. She's desperate to fit this together neatly; intent on making connections where none exist, building a picture and trying to convince other people of it. She's an expert at it, I've now come to realise.

She fixes me with a penetrating stare, willing me to believe. 'Listen. Samuel Cox and his family knew my family, okay?'

I play along. 'Okay.'

'So what if my mum wrote Sophie on the back of that photograph as a kind of alias? What if she had been taken into care and Samuel Cox had been visiting her, without Melanie knowing?'

'Edie, she didn't even go into the care home until after he took you, so it couldn't be her in that photo. They wouldn't have put her in a care home that far away either.'

Edie frowns. 'So it's not possible that Melanie Cox lied to me?'

'Sorry, Edes, I just don't buy it.'

'You don't think people are capable of lying?'

'Of course they're capable. But I say you forget Sophie and concentrate on what my father's up to.' I scan her face for a reaction and get nothing. 'Because I do buy that my father would go to any lengths to ruin us. You're avoiding that issue completely.'

I take her hand, but we both know I'm a big part of her problem. He's my father; it's my life he's trying to control. My future he is trying to influence. To him, Edie and her mother are collateral damage. If not for me, maybe she would have been left alone by him.

'I'm not avoiding it. I'm fully aware he wants me gone from your life.' Edie puffs her cheeks. 'And I know I'm clutching at straws with Sophie. But if Lisa turns out to be the spitting image of her, you've got a big apology to make.'

She slips her hand from mine, and I start the car. 'Listen, why don't we go for a drive? Have a pub lunch somewhere and talk it through properly?'

'Yeah. Can we go by Jaz's first though?' I want to talk to her, find out how she is. 'I was going to go tomorrow, but I can collect some of my stuff too. I guess I'm moving back in to our house, now your father won't be popping in any time soon?'

'Yeah. Thanks to Wilson, he knows we're back together anyway. Has Jaz taken your calls yet?'

'No. I tried her again last night, and she hung up on me. She only answers to tell me to leave her alone.'

'I can't believe your friendship has gone this sour.'

'I know, she's practically ghosting me. I'm worried about her. She's completely turned in on herself.' Edie stares out of the window. I can hardly hear her last sentence and don't even know whether I'm meant to. 'Jaz should have realised by now that I'm on her side.'

'Okay,' I tell her, feigning ignorance. 'We'll swing by. But I get to choose the pub afterwards.' I pull out of the car park onto Newton Road. In the stop-start Sandwell town traffic, Edie pulls out her phone and dials.

'Jaz, it's me. We're going to come by as we're in the area. I've got some news. Let me know if you're in.' She pauses. 'I've missed you, please talk to me.'

She cuts the call off with a frown.

'Still not answering?'

'No. It feels weird. She always had her phone glued to her and never let a call go to voicemail.'

I smile. According to Edie, even at work Jaz's phone was constantly poking out of the rear pocket of her scrubs, lighting up in the dark of night shifts, ringing at inappropriate moments, and often being answered as well. Apparently, Jaz once answered her phone when running to an arrest, guiding the crash trolley around corners with one hand, telling some guy she would call him back.

Edie hits redial. 'Jaz,' she calls into the phone. 'Jaa-aaz. Phone me back. Please.'

She waits, sucking her lip, then ends the call. Silently, she shakes her head at me. Nothing. Edie stares out of the window, brow furrowed. Although she never gave me details, she hinted once that Jaz has struggled in the past with depression, and sometimes still does. I can see all these thoughts in her eyes, just as I felt when I saw her note that morning she left. Just for a minute, you think the worst. Edie taps her phone screen again a couple of times.

'Matt, it's Edie. Yeah, have you heard anything from Jaz?' She pauses, listening. 'No, same here. Okay, thanks. I'll speak to you soon.' The worry is obvious in her eyes as she shuts the call down.

'What shall we do?' I ask.

Edie turns, decision made. 'Let's go over there.'

The drive through West Bromwich and Smethwick takes us half an hour, and we hit red at every set of temporary traffic lights and interchange. We skirt the grey, wind-whipped waters of Edgbaston reservoir, and cut down Monument Road. Jaz's flat is on the ground floor of Abbotts Court, a small, well-kept block of four in a large close. There are several similar blocks dotted around a park on the outskirts of a larger new-build estate. I park the car, and by the time I get to Jaz's flat Edie is already knocking on the door. We wait for a couple of minutes, then she tries again, harder. Not yet hammering, but not far off. I put my ear to the door. Inside, the flat is silent.

'She might be out?' I suggest.

'Look, the curtains are still drawn.'

'Where's your key?'

Edie rolls her eyes, frustrated. 'Back at the house.'

'Okay. What about checking the windows? It's warm, maybe she's left one open?'

Edie nods. My back and legs protesting, I wriggle through the bushes and over a fence onto the small patch of grass where her lounge window faces out. I try to look in, dipping and bobbing, but the curtains are closed. The flat has the feel of being abandoned.

'They're closed,' I call to her.

Across the patch of grass, Edie moves around the corner of the building towards where Jaz's bedroom window looks out over the car park. As she turns, even from where I stand the panic in her face is obvious. A moment later, she's back, shaking her head.

'They're closed too. Where is she?'

'What shall we do? Call the police?' I climb back over the fence, my funeral suit now scratched and dirty.

'We might have to. God, this isn't right, Harry. Something's wrong.'

'Look, don't panic.' I slip into my practical mode. 'Maybe nothing's happened. Maybe she got drunk and overslept. Maybe she has a guy in there?'

'Harry, I've known her answer her phone in the middle of sex, for God's sake.'

Her expression is tight, strained. I can't tell if she's being serious.

'Okay, let's check the door again.'

I knock hard, then kneel, peering through the letterbox. Along the hall is the front room, door slightly ajar. The open letterbox pulls a draught from the hall, carrying a stale, musty smell I can't quite place.

'Jaz,' I call, mouth pressed to the letterbox.

Edie kneels next to me, her face against mine. Her voice is shrill. 'Jaz?'

There is a small window next to the front door where the catch isn't fully engaged. Edie and I exchange a worried look; w*hat do you think?* She nods, and I work at the catch from below, trying to wiggle it loose. With the long flat surface of my car key pressed against the gap, I slide it past the PVC frame and against the catch. Infuriatingly slowly, it eases upwards. The key slips, the catch grazing my finger and leaving a streak of blood on the window.

'Shit.' I suck until the bleeding stops, then use my other hand. Finally, the catch gives and the window judders open, enough for me to kneel on the sill and reach down to open the larger window below. I pull myself through, falling against the door as I twist and drop.

The stale smell is stronger now, and there is an undertone of something else, as well.

Something organic, something bodily. Some primal instinct kicks in and my heart thuds. When I open the door, Edie pushes past, looking in the kitchen. My memory has finally located the smell. It has been a while for me, but all doctors recognise it eventually.

Reluctantly, I make my way to the front room. I don't want to see this, but I think I know what I'm going to find, and I want to spare Edie the horror of being the one who discovers her.

The first thing I see are her feet, poking out past the edge of the sofa as if she's sleeping on the floor. Her socks are on, but her slippers have come off and lie a few inches away. I step closer; I did clinical placements in my training, and I've seen bodies before, so I already know she's beyond help. The blood has pooled in her vessels and capillaries, drawn down by gravity, mottling the skin where she touches the floor. Jaz's lower legs are bare where her dressing gown has ridden up, and she is lying on her side, her arm splayed forward, as if she rolled off the sofa. Her long dark hair is now dull, covering her face, cheek down on her bright, patterned rug. I pull the throw from the sofa to cover her before Edie comes in. As I hear Edie's footsteps running towards me, I drape the blanket across Jaz's body. I don't want Edie seeing her like this.

Then her scream explodes in my ear as she pushes past me, skidding to her knees by Jaz's head, dragging the throw away again and pushing the hair away from her friend's face. Edie is frantic, feeling for a carotid pulse, resting her face against Jaz's, cheek to cheek, watching her chest, listening and feeling for breathing. She must know it's pointless; Jaz's lips are dark grey; her cheek mottled blue where it has been lying against the carpet. Her eyes are open, but dull. Opaque, like the patina on an ancient mirror. For the first time, I register the empty blister packs next to her on the floor. I can't make out what the medication is, but there are no spilled pills all around her like you'd see in the movies. She is a nurse; she knew how to do it properly.

I'm frozen, and time no longer exists. It is Edie's shout that pulls me out of it, a guttural roar of pain. Then she turns to me, her voice brittle and loud.

'For God's sake, Harry. Call an ambulance.'

My phone is in the car. I see Edie's on the floor next to her where she dropped it, and bend to grab it.

'What's the PIN?' She doesn't register, so I shout. 'Edie? The PIN?'

'Three-nine-seven-two,' she yells, rolling Jaz onto her back.

I'm flustered, it takes me a few seconds. Then I'm in.

I punch three nines on the keypad as Edie begins CPR, both of us knowing that, however quickly the ambulance gets here, it will still be far too late.

43

Edie

Where are the paramedics? We've called it in as a CPR in progress: why aren't they here yet?

My arms ache. As I push, her chest barely moves, her brown eyes stare beyond me into nothing. When Harry tries to help me, I shrug him away, carrying on as though she'll only be dead if I give up. He steps back, resting his hand on my shoulder briefly.

'I know she's gone, Harry, I know,' I shout.

But let me continue, let me work on, because this isn't right. This wasn't supposed to happen. It's not right that there's no life in her when there was always so much, when she was so vivid. It is not right that her body is cold; that the mottling of her skin shows how still the blood in her veins and arteries is, how still her heart is. It shouldn't be her. I don't care how long she's been here for, or when she took the pills. I want to keep going. Harry is looking at the blister pack, reading them out. Temazepam, prescribed to her on Tuesday. Two days after her suspension.

Then, blue lights are flashing on the walls where Harry has opened the curtains to let some light in. Feet are in the hall, voices, then hands are gently helping me away from the body. Their touch is kind, tender. They say comforting things to me. There are two female paramedics.

It's okay, love. We'll take over now. I'm so sorry.

I don't want to watch them pronounce her dead; don't want to see them connect their ECG monitor or see the asystole flat-line trace of her heart, which will show she is beyond resuscitation. They will fill in the details on their hand-held electronic records tablet, sign their forms, call the police, call the coroner. Then they will go on to their next job as if Jaz meant nothing.

Harry leads me to the kitchen and sits me on one of Jaz's mismatched chairs. I think out loud to him. *What were her last hours like? Did she wander the flat, unable to sleep? Did she take one Temazepam, two, three, and still not sleep? Did she want to sleep more than anything, enough to take them all?* He doesn't speak, but watches me ramble, filling the silence. I picture her crying, sobbing at the risk of losing the single thing she loved more than anything else in the world: her job.

I should have been here.

'Harry, why did you let me fall into this inertia, this denial?' I'm switching the blame, but I can't do otherwise. 'Why did I let you convince me to carry on as normal? Nothing is normal any more.'

'Edie, this wasn't my fault.'

Of course it wasn't him. I'm just turning on whoever's nearest. All of my clothes are still here in the spare bedroom, so I should have been staying with her, looking after her, not flitting home to be with Harry. More guilt to add to the rest. Harry puts his arm around me, then hands me back my phone. I'd forgotten he had it. One of the paramedics comes in, expressionless. This is all routine for her.

'We've covered her up, love, but we're going to have to leave her where she is I'm afraid.'

I follow her to the front room, avoiding looking at the covered mound in front of the sofa. The second paramedic is wandering around the flat, looking at Jaz's trinkets in a bored, intrusive way. She looks up as we come in. 'Sorry we couldn't do anything for her. Our control room is on to the police. They'll have to be notified as it's an unexpected death. Not that it looks suspicious, of course.'

'Are you going to wait on scene?' I manage.

She glances at her colleague, a chisel-faced woman in her forties. 'Yeah, we'll hold on until they arrive.'

'Thanks,' I say in a flat voice. Nothing is real, the whole thing is like some fevered hallucination. Harry's arm around my shoulder doesn't register, the white sheet with Jaz underneath it doesn't register.

'You okay?'

Harry rests his head against mine. It's a stupid question, but the only one that can be asked in these circumstances. What else do you say to someone? I nod and force a smile. I walk to the door of the spare bedroom, thinking about getting some of my clothes together to take with me, but I'm not ready. While the paramedics clear their equipment away, Harry checks the other rooms. I glance over his shoulder into her bedroom as he looks inside. Messy, as always. I return to the kitchen, fold my arms across the table and rest my head on them. When I close my eyes, the muted voices from the front room become distant and I let myself drift. A defence mechanism, perhaps? Close your eyes, and it all goes away.

Harry's voice pulls me from some dark, subterranean place. Not sleep, but not wakefulness either. The clock on the kitchen wall has moved three minutes while my eyes were shut.

'Edie, you need to see this.'

He has dropped something on the table. An A4 pad, filled with Jaz's writing.

'Where did you find this?'

'It was in her bedroom.'

Wiping my eyes, I study the pad. My own words come back to me; *write everything down, Jaz*. And she'd listened. There are jottings abut Morris, about Samuel Cox's diagnosis, his treatment. Pages of them. I scan the notes in her sloping, pointed handwriting. Some of the words are in capitals or underlined.

This Infusion Was CORRECT.
Morphine 1mg/ml. Double-checked.
NOT MY FAULT.

Her pen nearly went through the paper on the last one. I can picture her face pinched with anger, contorted with fury. As she wrote she would have been getting angrier, her knuckles white as she scrawled her innocence onto the page. I lay the pad out on the table and take a photo with my phone, noticing a jagged, half-glued edge along the top of the pad where a page has been torn out.

'What's this?'

'I don't know,' Harry replies. 'She must have ripped some pages out.'

'Or someone did?'

'Edes. Who else would have?'

I rub my eyes. 'You better put it back where you found it. This is something I want the police to see when they arrive too.'

Harry lifts the pad, reading it himself. 'She's written JC on here several times. That means my father, doesn't it?'

'Probably. We knew he'd visited Morris already.'

'Yes, but one of them is dated the day before the cardiac arrest.'

'Your father is tight with both Morris and Wilson. It won't prove anything.'

'Let's wait outside,' he says and sighs wearily. 'I can't stand to be in here any longer.'

It seems to take forever for the police to come. Eventually, a young constable with a wispy beard and a pink, scrubbed face arrives in a patrol car. He takes our names and asks us the standard questions. What time did you find her? Do you know her next of kin? I explain what happened, tell him about the suspension, tell him she left some notes. He nods sagely but isn't really listening. With an imperious air, he tells us we're free to go, and they will be in touch if needed. We are dismissed.

In the car we don't speak for several minutes. Harry turns the engine on and stares at the ambulance pulling away.

'How could she have done that to herself, Edie?'

'You read her notes. You don't mistake fentanyl for morphine. It just doesn't happen.'

'None of this is right, is it?'

'Listen, Harry, I'm going to see if I can contact Lisa Saunders tomorrow. The woman Trevor told us about. She's Samuel Cox's daughter, so I'm going to ask her if she will see me. I want closure on that, at least.'

Finally, he nods. 'Okay. But I'm worried, Edes. I know my father better than anyone in this world, and something scares me about this whole thing.'

241

'Your father wouldn't hurt you, Harry. You're his blue-eyed boy.'

'It's not me I'm scared for.'

'You don't think he's finished with me, do you?'

He shakes his head, *no*. Then he looks across the car park to where the young policeman has just emerged from Jaz's flat. 'Not by a long way.'

44

Edie

Lisa Saunders' house suggests she's been coping with life better than her mother. I'd punched the postcode she'd given me into my phone, and the grating satnav voice has guided me along the M6 to the M1, then off near Milton Keynes towards a village called Stony Stratford. I arrive just after eleven on Saturday morning, having slept for less than an hour. Every time I closed my eyes, the sight of Jaz, twisted and mottled on the carpet, filled the darkness. Whatever thoughts I had of riding this out, seeing it through and then moving on, vanished as soon as I saw her body.

The cottage I'm now parked outside is detached, rustic, and reclines prettily in an established, immaculately re-wilded garden. The cottage is double-fronted, and recently renovated with new sash windows, fresh pointing on the chimney, an obviously new front door. The heavy, brass knocker thuds deeply, masking the noise of my pulse throbbing in my head. I take a few calming breaths through pursed lips. I had called Lisa the day before, using the number Trevor Cox had given me, and it was only when I mentioned his name that she believed who I was. There had been long silences on the phone, several of them long enough to make me think she'd ended the call.

The door swings open. The man in front of me is tall and handsome in a square-jawed, standard sort of way. Not my type; I go for the quirkier, more complicated guys like Harry. Behind him is a flagstone hallway with wooden stairs sweeping upwards and a pine door, half open, where the sound of young children shouting and laughing floats from the kitchen.

At last I find my voice. Too late to go back now. 'I'd like to speak to Lisa, please.'

'Are you Edie?'

'Yeah. I'm a friend of her Uncle Trevor.'

'She was crying yesterday. Your call shocked her.'

He looks like he is caught between letting me in and slamming the door. I garble an excuse. 'I'm sorry. I really am. I wouldn't have called, but I have to speak to her. I couldn't do it over the phone.'

He pauses, then opens the door a little wider. 'I suppose. She said you were coming. Look, I'm going to stay out of the way, all right?'

He studies me a moment longer, then beckons me in. I step inside, and he pads down the hallway into the kitchen. He shushes the children's voices and emerges with a blonde two-year-old girl in his arms, bouncing her up and down. The small girl waves shyly at me as he takes her upstairs. A few steps behind them, a woman in jogging bottoms and a jumper comes towards us across the flagstone tiles. Lisa. I don't recognise her, but people change, don't they? The silence drags for several uncomfortable seconds.

'You'd better come into the lounge.'

For the first ten minutes she doesn't speak as I embark on a stream-of-consciousness babbling, convinced she is going to either scream for help, throw me out or call the police. Although I had told her who I was and why I wanted to speak to her, the atmosphere still feels like it could flip either way. I keep talking as her frown deepens, before finally explaining what had happened with Samuel Cox. If what Trevor said is true and mother and daughter are estranged, then Melanie wouldn't have told her about my visit, and this would all be new to her. I wait for the shock to sink in, leaning forward, keeping my expression neutral. Her eyes shine as tears form, but she remains composed.

She pulls a crumpled tissue from her pocket and dabs her eyes quickly and efficiently.

'So you think my dad got himself admitted to your intensive care on purpose?'

'I don't think, Lisa. I know. I watched him on CCTV outside the hospital.'

'Why have you come here?' she asks bluntly. 'I haven't seen my father for twenty years. I haven't seen my mother for nearly that long, either. I've made a life for myself here, as you can probably see. I don't want any of my family upset by this.'

'I promise that's not my intention. I just want to know what you remember. Trevor said you were in foster care.'

She nods. 'My mother couldn't cope. I couldn't cope either. I became… difficult, I suppose. But that's not to say I didn't partly blame her for what he did.'

'Did you ever try to contact her? After you were put in care?'

'Yes, but at first, she didn't want anything to do with me. Apparently, I reminded her of him. After that, I didn't want anything to do with her in return. I had a good long-term foster home, Edie. It wasn't as difficult an upbringing as many kids in care have. At least not physically, my foster parents were good people. Emotionally…' She pauses, puffing her cheeks. She is a woman used to keeping things in, I recognise it instantly. We're not so different. 'Well, emotionally, it was obviously hard because of what had happened.'

'I'm sorry for putting you through this, but I sometimes feel like I'm going crazy not knowing. In the last few weeks I've genuinely feared for my…' I tail off, conscious that I'm oversharing. Why am I telling a woman I've only just met I'm worried for my sanity? In the middle of the silence that follows, I hear myself voicing the question that has been on my lips since I arrived. 'Lisa, what care homes were you in?'

She shakes her head. 'Only one. I was lucky, I was placed quite quickly.'

'Were you ever in the southwest?'

'No, it was Cambridgeshire. Why?'

'Never mind.' Harry was right, of course it wouldn't have been her. I pass the photograph across to her. 'Do you recognise the girl standing next to me on this photograph?'

She studies it, shrugs and passes it back. 'Is she your sister?'

'I don't know.' A sudden wave of tiredness sweeps over me. Lisa tilts her head in concern.

'Are you okay?'

'Yeah, these last few days have just been…' I pause as the feel of Jaz's cold skin comes back to me, the stale, sickly air of the flat. I drag my hands across my eyes. 'They've been difficult. Horrible. Just over a month ago, my life was ordinary. Boring, almost. I liked it that way.'

As I blurt out my feelings to this woman who I've met today for the first time, our eyes meet, and there is a connection so strong it stuns me. She senses it too, she must do, because she comes over to the sofa and sits next to me, so close we are touching.

'Edie, I'm so sorry for you.'

'Thank you,' I tell her. She has as much to be upset about as I do, and I try to pull myself together. I came here not knowing whether I would tell her Samuel was innocent, but now I know I never will, just like I'll never tell Trevor either, despite my promise to myself. The damage is already done; there is no repairing it. I can't pile more guilt into their lives; I don't want them to have any more regrets than they already do. But I still want to know more about her. I want to know how she feels. 'Lisa, would you be prepared to tell me about your father? Your childhood?'

'I can tell you some things, but, like you, a lot of it is hazy.' She sighs, as if she is about to being a long, difficult journey. 'What I can tell you for certain is I hate my father with every fibre of my being. You say you've talked to my mother?'

'Yes.' I nod. 'You probably know, she hates him too.'

'Not like I do. But she might have told you already. About the affairs?'

'Yes, she mentioned that.'

'I think my mother, for all her faults, loved him deeply. But she would scream and cry to herself when he was not home, because she knew he was with another woman. She thought she knew who the woman was, but time must have clouded everything for her by now. Years ago, she would have been all too willing to blurt her accusations out. I used to listen to her in the kitchen, yelling curses at him and the bitch he was with.'

'Who was she?'

'A local woman. I don't know how they met. Every time he left the house, there was a torrent of accusations, then tears after he'd gone, because my mother felt so guilty and hurt. Torturing herself with the hope she was wrong. But inside, she always knew she was right about him, and because of that, as a seven-year-old, I knew as well, and my hate grew. I used to lie awake at night in bed, crying silently, wishing for him to leave for good. I didn't expect my wish to come true in the way it did. We all carry guilt, don't we?'

'Do you know the woman's name? The affair?'

She thinks for a moment, a second that stretches into eternity. Eventually the word sinks into me, as if it had always been there. 'Jenny.'

Jenny. How much hatred must she have had to let her ex-lover rot in prison? How much shame?

Lisa is still talking, lost in the past. 'The family had fractured irreparably by that time. We never went on holiday together, but he would go off for a week every summer, pretending it was with his friends on a hill-walking holiday or something. My mother knew it was with this woman.'

The writing on the photograph. Hers. I count my breathing to slow it down. 'How long did this affair go on for?'

'I don't know, I was young. It probably went on for years. We felt abandoned. And then, when he was convicted, my mum abandoned me too. I think she thought I was tainted or something, that's how it felt. She never loved me the same way after she realised what was happening. After she discovered he'd had a child with this other woman.'

'A child?' My voice is little more than a hoarse whisper. 'Samuel Cox had a child from the affair?'

'A daughter. I heard my mother screaming at him about it.'

'He had a daughter with Jenny?'

'Yes, in nineteen ninety-five.'

I feel as if I'm about to throw up. That's why Cox performed the abduction. That's why he risked everything, why he suffered years in prison. Took all the abuse they could dish out.

'So he did it to protect me,' I whisper. 'He felt like he had to do something.'

She leans forward to hear. 'Protect you?'

It is why he accused Michael, it is why I felt nothing but love when I remembered the beach, nothing but safety when I went back to the coast. It's why he was so desperate to keep a young, traumatised girl safe. A girl who everyone else thought was a stranger to him. To the rest of the world, this looked like a random abduction. But it wasn't. It was an act of deep, enduring love.

'Edie, are you okay?'

'Lisa, I'm Jenny's only child.' I lapse into silence. It drags on, neither of us looking at each other. When I speak, my voice is a low, incredulous whisper. 'Samuel Cox was my father.'

45

Harry

'How can you stay so calm? Didn't you hear me? I'm Samuel Cox's daughter.' Edie is pacing the kitchen, her food untouched. 'Lisa Saunders' half-sister.'

How she drove home in the state she's in, I'll never know. She'd phoned me from Buckinghamshire, barely coherent, then since she came through the door her conversation has been a non-stop monologue.

I immediately knew my father would have already got this information from Jenny. That he already knows everything Edie does. The fact he's biding his time makes me more nervous than ever. I think of him working on Jenny, providing her with just enough sedative to lower her guard, not quite enough to make her incoherent. He was in clinical practice for years, he'll know exactly what he's doing in terms of doses. The depth of the deception that Jenny has constructed intrigues me; and it'll intrigue him, too. Edie's mother would make a case study that would get him on the front cover of the *British Journal of Psychiatry*. For her to have had this level of denial all these years is quite remarkable. To keep the truth hidden for as long as Jenny has, and to harbour such loathing towards the man who apparently tried to save her daughter, is a fascinating pathology of revenge. And if she's not motivated by pure hatred, then what a secret she must be hiding to keep a man in prison all those years rather than let the truth out.

Edie is watching me. 'Harry, are you listening?'

'Of course,'

'It explains why Samuel Cox would have gone through so much

pain and trauma for me. How could Melanie Cox let it happen? My mother too?'

I sit next to her. 'Edes, revenge is all some people have got. You don't understand how deep some people's anger goes.'

'No, I don't. But both women wanting to punish him? What did he do to deserve that?

'You'd have to ask your mother.'

Her expression hardens. 'That evil bitch. Why would she start telling me the truth now? She's already spilled everything to your bloody father. She told him first. She was the one who told him about the fact I thought Sophie drowned.'

'You don't know that for sure, Edes.'

She stares at me. 'Yes, I do. And that's why your father visited the coast. He wants to know what happened. And my mother is…' She fills her lungs and exhales loudly. 'She's fucking helping him.'

'Come on, Edes.'

'I can't remember though, Harry. I think…' the words are thick and slow '… I think I watched Sophie drown. What if I could have helped her? What if my mother knows? She's talked to him.'

'Okay, but only because he's got her doped to the eyeballs. You saw that yourself. Anyway, guilt makes people do strange things. Don't you see, people with guilty secrets *want* to talk. Why do you think Melanie Cox saw you, then cut you off? Why did she give you his diary?'

Our eyes lock. 'Because she had torn herself apart over the years. She felt she owed me that much.'

'Right. Guilt. Your mother just processed it in a different way, that's all.'

'Don't make excuses for her, Harry. Samuel Cox was my real father.' Her mouth is drawn into a tight, angry slit. 'And now he's dead. Do you think someone meant to kill him?'

'No. Who would have? And how?'

We lapse into an uneasy silence, but my mind drifts back to Michael Carter. What if Carter knew that Edie wasn't his? What if he knew, every time he did whatever horrible things he did to her, that he was getting his own sick form of revenge on Samuel Cox? It makes sense. Michael had been made to look a fool for years. Cuckolded. If he knew about the affair all along, is it so hard to believe he would torture Edie? Abuse her, if he chose to? How better to get revenge on a person than make their child suffer? As I watch Edie staring at the table, picking at her thumb, I wrestle with my conscience. A thought that had occurred to me when she first arrived home won't leave me alone. It has morphed from a throwaway thought into something sinister. I need to tell her about it and take the consequences.

'Edie, there's something else. I mean it's just speculation.'

'Haven't I got enough on my plate?'

'This is something we need to discuss. Don't take this the wrong way, but when you came in a moment ago it occurred to me what a ground-breaking case study your mother would make. What incredible raw material she would provide for research on the power of repression and denial. The power of revenge and transference. For a thesis on a form of acquired psychopathy, where guilt has damaged the empathic response.'

'What are you talking about, Harry? My mother and I aren't bloody case studies.'

'I know.' I pause, not sure whether to carry on or let it drop. It's just speculation, a horrible, nightmarish theory, but now it's there I can't ignore it, and I need to make her aware of the possibility. I need to plant the seed, and there's no going back if I do. 'But what if that's exactly how my father sees you both? Now he's got you where he wants you?'

'What do you mean?'

'You and your mother. Case studies.'

'No.' Incredulous, she stands and paces to the worktop, shaking her head. Her dark hair swishes against her shoulder with the force of her denial. 'No way.'

The possibility has hit a nerve, but I have to carry on, even though I know I'm hurting her. 'Seriously. I know how his mind works. It'd be like a bonus for him, a permanent reminder to him of his own authority. He splits us up, and this would be the cherry on top as far as he is concerned; he gets to study you both. You and your mother would be his little project. He'll get a feature in the *British Journal*. Conference papers, you name it.'

'That's impossible.'

'Why? How do you think people make their names if not through specific cases? Kim Peek, Anna O, Little Albert? When I found the file on you in his study, it had articles on dissociation, repression, intergenerational trauma. Familial co-dependency. He was thinking about you and your mother, Edie.'

'No, no, no. Harry.' Her head is still shaking, trying to throw the thought away, but the tone of rising panic in her voice is unmistakable. 'He wouldn't be able to get away with it, would he?'

'Edie, once you're in his institution, once you're in his secure unit, he can get away with whatever he likes.'

'No, he is still accountable to other people.'

'Patients in institutions have no agency, Edes. No power. I've seen it myself, all my career. You've seen the news reports; this stuff goes on even in care homes, for God's sake. Think about it: once you're both in there, who then believes you over him? Who believes a psychiatric patient?'

'Oh God. I couldn't stand it.' She turns and shuffles back to the table in shock. Her eyes are wet. She sits down again and sinks her head onto the table. 'Harry, what do we do?'

I put my arm across her shoulder and move closer. She flinches momentarily, uncertain, but I hold her there tightly, pulling her into me. Keeping her there. I kiss her head, lean my own against it.

'We're not done yet,' I whisper. 'I've been thinking about how to deal with him. My father's reputation is the key to this. He's vain, he's a narcissist. He's a bully. He's all those things and more. He's bullied me my whole life, made it a misery. But when that happens, you learn to recognise the person's moods, their methods. I know his weak spot.'

'What, other than he's a complete bastard?'

'No, actually he sees that as a strength.'

252

Edie rests her head in her hands, and, in the middle of the tension, we both laugh, just for a few seconds. The laughter is bitter, but it's enough to get her to raise her head, meet my eyes and engage with me again.

'Seriously, you have no idea how conceited he is,' I say as our smiles fade. 'His reputation is everything to him. It's why everything he's done so far is so underhand, so hard to pin anything on. Proof is everything, he knows that. He wants you to react; it's why I stopped you confronting him the night Samuel Cox died. We need to see your mother; document the treatment he's been giving her. If we can get proof, we can build a case, something that would damage his reputation if we made it public, and then we've got him. That's the way to protect ourselves.'

'I wish I'd managed to photograph her medication sheet last time,' she whispers, then grabs my arm, hopeful. 'Maybe I can persuade my mother to tell the truth about him? I can record her on my phone. We need to speak to her again, quickly. I'll go Monday.'

'You need more than oral testimony, and it's unlikely she'll talk anyway. I'll meet you there. I'll come and play the indignant psychiatrist. You know, pull rank, ask to see files and so on.'

'No.' She is emphatic. 'That will just raise the alarm. I want to make it a simple visit.'

'Okay, but if there's any trouble I can be there in an hour.'

'What about your father though? He'll know.'

'Not until it's too late. He's in London. He has a conference at Imperial College this week. I relented and spoke to my mother recently. She's desperate for us two to reconcile; she tells me everything.'

She frowns, chewing her thumb. 'Are you sure he'll be away?'

'Yes, I'm certain. By eight Monday morning, my father will be on the train. My mother practically gave me his schedule. Even if Claydon Manor reached him on the train and he turned around, you would be gone before he came back.' She flashes me an uncertain look and I shake my head. 'I know what you're thinking, but don't worry. He won't come back, because it would look bad if he didn't show in London. But what do we say to Claydon Manor?'

She straightens. 'That my mother's brother has died, and we need to break the news to her. It's an emergency, right?'

'She doesn't have a brother. You told me you and her had no close relatives.'

'They're not to know that, are they?'

She exhales heavily, a full, determined breath. Having a plan has dispersed the fog of anxiety for both of us. As I look at her, I'm flooded with gratitude for the way she trusts me. Why doesn't she hate me like she hates him? I can't answer that, but I'm glad. No, more than glad; I'm elated she doesn't think I'm like him.

But Jesus, what dysfunctional families we come from. What strange families, full of liars and deceivers. And here we are, Edie and I; the two of us, who somehow found each against all the odds. Who met and fell in love even though we were mired in a network of other people's denial, lost amongst so many others who were hiding their true selves away. Was how we met really a coincidence? Was it random, or were we drawn together? If I believed in fate, then I would also believe that two young people with such maladjusted families must recognise something in each other. And when they do, won't the connection hit them both like a surge of electricity? Yes, it must be true, because I know now, whatever happens, that we are inseparable. I'm never letting her go.

And there is only one way we are getting out of this together. One way we can give my father what he deserves.

It's a long shot but, after this, we might be free of him.

46

Edie

I've been parked in a corner of the grounds for the last half an hour, watching Claydon Manor from afar. There is the day unit on the left side of the building, where people come for various therapies; a small theatre suite for ECT day patients; the voluntary inpatient wing, where people pay to get their various anxieties, paranoias and phobias treated. And just beyond, rising above the two arms of the building, is the main house, where the secure unit holds the people who – for whatever reason – aren't allowed to leave. That's the building my mother is currently incarcerated in. Is that a strong word, incarcerated? No, that's exactly what it is.

I'd called at eight-thirty and, after a terse exchange, Sue Willard had reluctantly agreed to my visit. But as soon as the phone was down, I knew, the senior sister would be informing Creighton, and I drove the twenty-five miles to Claydon Manor praying Harry was right and she'd be unable to get hold of him. Over the years, this institution has become a spectre hovering at the edge of my life. I hate its walls, its windows, its fake normality. It is a monster crouching in the pretty green foliage of the English countryside. As I took the familiar roads, my mother's voice echoed in my ears, getting louder. '*f you're not careful, you'll be in here with me.* There we will sit, she and I, dull-eyed and medicated. Getting older day by day, never to be released.

But my confidence has grown as I've been watching the house. James Creighton isn't here; his car isn't in the car park, and the building just *feels* safe. I can't rationalise it, but I know he's not here. I'd tried to get my sixth sense working when I'd rung at eight-thirty, and told Sue Willard I would need to see my mother in person to deliver some bad news. Willard's voice was laced with the icy hostility I'd come to expect and, what's worse, she has the habit of long phone silences, which encourage people to babble and confess all. She and James Creighton are a professional match made in hell. But although there was a hint of distaste, as if she was talking to some deeply unsavoury human being, I didn't sense any overt threat.

'This highly irregular, Doctor Carter,' Willard says as she greets me at the reception. 'But given it's a bereavement in the family, I suppose we can make an exception.'

'She would want to hear this from me, Sue. So kind of you to accommodate it.' I just about keep the sarcasm out of my voice. 'You know how she can get sometimes.'

I follow her through the metal door to the unit, which clicks shut behind me as the automatic lock engages. I've walked straight into the maw of the beast, and am dependent upon this nasty woman to release me when the time comes. Thankfully, she doesn't notice my discomfort. We pass through another heavy door, and she leads me past the day room. I pause, chest pounding. 'Where are we going?'

Willard smiles blandly. 'Your mother is in her bedroom. She's tired today.'

Tired? Drugged, you mean.

I fight my anxiety. I'm being led further and further on into the heart of the secure wing. I know about institutions, and I'm used to them, but only on my terms. Harry's words are ringing around my head. *Don't worry, Edes, he can't be contacted.* But what if Harry's wrong? What if Willard is leading me straight to Creighton, and some trumped-up diagnosis? How would they phrase it in the notes? Edie Carter is delusional, hysterical; she requires observation, assessment, a forty-eight-hour period of monitoring. We authorise her to be held under Section Two. And here's the horrible thought making my heart race: the more I protest, the angrier I get, the more I yell and scream, the more proof I give them. The more ammunition. Once you've been admitted to these places, how do you go about proving yourself rational?

For a moment, I doubt Harry. The only person I've come to rely on in my life is myself, and my default position is that other people can't be trusted. But Harry was always different, I remind myself. He *can* be trusted. From the moment I met him when I started sessions at the King George, there was something about him I connected with. I sensed that the reason he was interested in finding out more about me, about what made me tick, was because of the way he felt about his own life. There was something deep in him too, which matched something buried in me, and I have never been able to fully explain what it was. A sort of emptiness, or a lack of something to anchor ourselves to. A vacuum that other young people didn't seem to have.

So as I walk along the corridor behind Sue Willard, her white shoes squeaking on the lino, I wrestle with a growing, gnawing anxiety. What if I was wrong? What if Harry and his father have been toying with me? Then Willard is ushering me into a room and there she is, slumped in an armchair, her back to the window. It's the first time I've seen her in the secure unit bedroom. It looks like a tired budget hotel. A single bed in the corner is neatly made, with three books strewn across it. There is a book propped open in her lap but she's not reading it; her eyes are fixed on the floor, distant and dreaming.

Willard flashes an insincere smile at me. 'Please don't upset your mother this time, Doctor Carter.' Without waiting for a reply, she leaves.

When the door has clicked shut, I sit on the bed opposite her. Her eyes wander from the floor to my face, glazed and vacant, studying me but not seeing me.

'Mum, it's Edie.'

At my name, she smiles. Her eyes drift to the wall, her voice is a quiet drawl. 'Edie. You've come back.'

I get my phone ready, scroll to the voice recorder, press record.

There is no time for niceties. No time to break this to her gently. 'Mum, I need you to be honest with me. I forgive you for those lies you told me last time. But you've been lying to me all my life. Now

I want the truth. Tell me everything about what's happened to you here.'

'No one's been lying.'

'Yes, Mum. You have. I know I'm Samuel Cox's daughter.'

Her gaze searches my face, seeing me properly for the first time. Her thin, pinched lips mouth the words, roll the sound of his name around. *Samuel Cox.* Her mouth forms an uncomprehending circle, and then the sides of her mouth drop in a frown so desperately sad it makes me want to cry. She stares at a point between my eyes, as if trying to gaze into my thoughts, into the essence of me.

'Samuel?'

'Mum, what has James Creighton got you on?' She frowns, and I put the phone closer to her. 'Tell me what they've been doing to you?'

Her thought processes feel infuriatingly slow, but there is no anger in her tone now, just a deep, bitter-sweet regret. A nostalgia for something she can't quite grasp any more. Then her eyes are distant again, vacant. She won't look at me. 'I loved Sam, Edie.'

'Yes, Mum, I believe you.'

'Those summers were the best times we have ever had.'

'Mum, listen. I need you to talk to me. I haven't got long. I need to find out whether James Creighton has been abusing his position to get information on us. I need proof. What medication has he given you?'

'And Sam loved you both, you know. Why were you so jealous of her?'

'Mum, I don't care about the past, I care about now. Talk, please.'

She continues to ignore me, smiling at a memory long gone. Her eyes shine brighter, as if something has pushed its way through the fog. 'We were all running away. It couldn't last forever, could it?'

Then she looks at me as she used to when I was younger, and the phone on the table is forgotten. For one precious moment, it is just me and her, deep in each other's eyes for once. She is so frail, I can see her shoulder blades jutting through her jumper. I know the look of someone who has stopped eating, I recognise someone who has given up. I reach over and turn the voice recorder off. She won't say anything, and, even if she did, it wouldn't mean anything. It wouldn't be admissible. I just want this one moment to last, her and me, connecting. One moment for her to say what we did was all right. One instant where we can forgive ourselves for what we've done to each other.

'Mum? I love you so much.'

As I speak, she stares at me again and her face becomes animated, but it is not with the love I'd hoped for. It's no longer regret in her eyes, or remembrance, or bitter-sweet nostalgia.

It is deep, undiluted fury.

'You love me?' Her voice is shrill, harsh. Hate-filled. 'You *love* me?'

And then she is on me. She moves so quickly I can't even get out of my chair. Whatever drug-induced mist she was lost in has evaporated and she is a malign spirit, her hair flying, her eyes bright. She straddles me and holds my head, her nails digging in behind my ears, pushing as if she wants to tear my face off. Her eyes are inches from mine, her breath is cloying.

'You love me?' she hisses. 'Well, my precious girl, you should know by now that I hate *you*.'

The door flies open, and two porters come in. How did they react so quickly? It is only then, as they grab one of my mother's arms each, that I notice the small black dome on the ceiling, shining in the corner. CCTV. I'm grateful that Sue Willard wasn't one of the staff who responded, but I know it will get back to Creighton anyway. The young porters ease my mother off me and look at us both as if their pay grade doesn't cover this kind of stuff. My pulse rushes in my ears, pounding in my throat. I try to find my voice but can only manage a low moan. The taller porter has his hand on my shoulder, and I shrug it off.

'I'm fine,' I say eventually, although my voice is shaking. I look at the woman who raised me, who used to love me. She has fallen back onto the bed. She fixes me with a dull stare, then beckons me toward her. I lean in, wary, but the fight has gone out of her eyes now.

'It's too late for you, my girl.'

'What do you mean?'

'He knows,' she hisses. 'He knows it all.'

'Mum, what have you told him?'

'Everything. I'm here forever.' She smiles, a lost, sad smile. 'And now you're next.'

47

Edie

When I get back to the reception, Sue Willard is behind the desk. She watches me as I buzz through and keep walking, staring straight ahead. Shafts of yellow morning sun slant through the main glass door, ten metres in front of me, and onto the reception carpet. The green of the trees and the blue of the sky suck me towards them across the reception area. I want to be out of here more than I've ever wanted anything in my life. The woman who used to be my mother is lost to me now, the web of lies that has held us together for all of these years has been ripped apart. Once I'm through the door, I'm never coming back. My legs are like jelly, waves of nausea are sweeping through my stomach.

Then Sue Willard's measured, rational voice stops me. 'Doctor Carter? Could you wait a moment please?'

I keep moving, but the green LED light next to the main door flicks red. She has locked it. I swivel and meet her expressionless eyes. 'Could you open the door please?'

'We'd like to speak to you a moment.'

A movement in the far corner of the reception draws my attention. Kieran has appeared from a door behind the desk. Sue Willard glances at him.

'What's going on?' I ask, keeping my composure, allowing a tone of clinical authority into my voice. A tone I'm desperate for them to respond to.

'We want to speak about what just happened in the room,' Willard replies. Only then do I see the bank of small monitors along the reception desk. There's the bedroom; she is sitting in her chair again, motionless. Seeing that I've noticed the monitors, Willard smiles politely. 'So, as I said, do you have a few minutes?'

My head is shaking, too emphatic. 'No. I'm sorry, but I need to go, I'm in a hurry.'

'It won't take long.'

I rest my hands on the top of the counter and lean across. Attack is the best form of defence, so I fix my gaze on her glacial eyes. 'First, I'd like to know why my mother is so heavily sedated. What have you done?'

Willard smiles her robotic smile. 'It's because she's been agitated. As you've just seen. Her sedatives have been prescribed.'

'And I know by who,' I sneer. 'I suppose you've told Professor Creighton I'm here?'

Her smile doesn't falter. 'He asked to be notified of visitors to Mrs Carter, yes.'

'And you managed to get hold of him, did you?'

'I'm not at liberty to say.' The smile fades, cools further by a degree or two. Kieran moves closer, his brow furrowed.

'Let me see my mother's records.'

'You know we can't do that.' Her voice is monotone.

Claustrophobia is sucking the oxygen from me, I'm being smothered in her dead, cloying, inflexible manner. 'Okay. Well, you listen to me, you fucking bitch. You open that door right now, or I'm calling the police.'

She takes a step back and frowns. 'You can't speak to me like that.'

Something inside me has snapped, and I no longer have the willpower to restrain myself. I am playing right into Creighton's hands, but somehow all those years of my lost life have sprung to the front of my mind and the injustice is crippling my sense of reason. They don't understand me, they don't understand the woman imprisoned in their institution either, the woman who protected me all those years. They don't understand either of us. And I won't let them do this to me.

'You can tell Creighton I'm on to him.' My voice comes from

miles away, as if it is someone else's. 'You can tell him I know what he's up to.'

Sue Willard's voice pierces the moment. 'Oh, I'll tell him everything, Doctor Carter.'

She reaches for the phone, and my focus is back again, as sharp and bright as a razor. I'm quicker than her, and, before she can dial, I've snatched the receiver from her hand and dropped it back in its cradle.

'Call him when I'm gone.' I hold her level, icy gaze. 'And when you do, tell him I'm going to make sure the world knows who he is and exactly what he's done. I'll ruin him. You tell him I will fight every inch of the way. You tell him that, okay?' Kieran moves to her side, eyes fixed on me. He is not sure what to do, as I stare at Sue Willard, daring her to defy me. 'Now, you open that fucking door.'

The breeze is wonderful against my flushed, burning cheeks. I run to the car even though I should walk; I don't care that running looks even more suspicious. As I get in the car, glancing back at Claydon Manor and its grey stone walls, all I see is the might of all the institutions I've ever known. All I can feel is their implacable power. How pointless my words to Sue Willard were. How empty. Helplessness and fear washes over me. What power do I have?

I get my phone out; shit, I'm on five per cent. I used Harry's charger last night because mine is at Jaz's, so how can the battery be dead? Staring at the red power icon, I call Harry, desperate to speak to him. In the shadow of Claydon Manor everything is unravelling, and I need to get away. I need time to evaluate the situation, time to breathe. To be with someone I don't feel threatened by. I need to plan what to do; to try to find a way to turn this around. The vision of Jaz, lying still and blue on the floor, comes back to me and my breath see-saws, too fast. My hands begin tingling, I'm hyperventilating.

Questions. Questions.

What does Creighton know? He thinks I'm crazy, right?

Is it all over?

Harry's phone rings out. *Oh for fuck's sake Harry, where are you? I need you.*

Please leave a message after the beep.

I force my breathing to slow down.

'Harry. It's Edie. Please ring me back as soon as you get this. I need to talk.' I suck in air, collecting my racing thoughts. My composure has deserted me. 'My mother is in a bad way, Harry. She's told everything to your father, and I'm not going to get anything from her.' More breaths. 'Harry, I need to speak to you. Willard tried to keep me at Claydon Manor, but I got out. Meet me at Jaz's flat. I'm going there to get the rest of my things. Meet me there as soon as you can, okay? I'm scared.' A last sentence before I ring off, desperate, pleading.

'I want us to get away from here.'

48

Harry

I get out of the shower to hear my phone ringing downstairs. As the ringtone jingles, I pogo one-legged across the bedroom floor, pulling my boxer shorts on as I go. I run out of the bedroom towel-drying my hair, then stop and listen on the landing. Silence; it has stopped. I wait, but it doesn't ring again. I'm hoping Edie will have spoken to Jenny by now, and I'm desperate to find out how it went. I rush to get dressed, then head downstairs. At the foot of the stairs I stop, immediately wary. The front door, which was pushed fully closed, is now on the latch. Dragging my memory, I try to place the faint lingering smell of cologne in the hall. Recognition hits me in seconds. It's his.

My hand freezes on the banister newel, one foot still on the stairs. I'm like a startled cat, listening for noises. The movement of shoes on the flagstone floor reaches me; he is in the kitchen. So much for the London lunch and the Imperial College conference. Mum couldn't tell a lie to save her life, and she was convinced he was going down there, so he must have delivered an Oscar-worthy performance. The sandalwood of the cologne clogs my nostrils, a fragrance that threaded through my childhood. My father is a creature of habit.

My anger rising, tempered by a slow burning sense of panic, I push the kitchen door open. There he is, standing at the breakfast bar, leaning on it as if he owns the place. My phone lies near the fruit bowl where I left it. His eyes follow me across the kitchen as I check the phone log.

One missed call. Edie.

'How long have you been here?'

265

'That's a fine way to greet your father.'

'Did you hear this ring?'

'I've only just got here.'

My tone is terse, to the point. 'How did you get in?'

'You left the door on the latch, Harry. Thank you. Not very security-conscious, though.'

I grab my phone and check Find My. Edie is driving away from Claydon Manor. We might still be okay. I move closer to my father, phone in hand, until we're a couple of feet apart. A faint smile lurks in his eyes, a relaxed, *I-am-in-control* smirk. I know exactly what he's planning.

'You expected to find me at work and Edie here, didn't you?'

'Yes, naturally. It would have been much simpler, Harry. Never mind, we'll do it the hard way.'

In a moment of clarity, I see straight through his methods of control. People fall for it; they *want* to fall for it. Most people like to be told what to do, they like to be controlled. What else explains why no one is prepared to stand up to him, call him out? He has Morris in his pocket. Wilson too. I've heard how he controls the council at the Royal College, how he dishes out favours or withholds them to buttress his power, playing the political game. Toxic leadership *par excellence*. He has fooled me with it for most of my life, but not any longer. I've now made my own decisions for what *I* want. I'm just as clever as he is, and he will soon find out that I'm able to make the big calls too.

I've had enough of being around him. I want him out of my life forever. I push him towards the door. 'Get out.'

'Harry, you know you can't stop this now. You can't help her any more.'

'I said get out,' I yell, pushing him towards the front door. He straightens his jacket and opens the door.

'Enough with all the bravado, Harry. Stop playing this game. You're not stupid, you know exactly what's going on.'

'Fuck you. I hope I never see you again.'

The words sound peevish, childish. Emotion delivered by a

hammy actor. He smiles knowingly, then turns. 'Son, I'm right. And you'll thank me for what I'm going to do.'

I slam the door behind him. As soon as I'm back in the kitchen, I call the voicemail number on my phone and put it on speaker.

You have no new messages and five saved messages.

No new messages? There were four saved messages before, ones I hadn't got around to deleting. Now there are five. That means Edie left a message when she rang, and it has already been listened to.

By my father. The lying bastard. I slam the phone down on the worktop, cursing myself for leaving it unlocked.

I play the most recent message back. She sounds distraught, panicking. *Meet me at Jaz's.*

Then I remember the phone tracker. My fingers fumble with the app, but she doesn't appear on it. Her phone is off. I call her anyway: no answer. Straight to voicemail.

Come on, Edie.

I leave a message, then run up the stairs two at a time and throw some things into a bag; a change of clothes, a few toiletries, the charger. Of course, the charger.

The faulty charger I gave Edie to use on her phone last night.

Back downstairs, I run to the hook in the kitchen next to the fridge-freezer, where the keys are. Fobs and keyrings scatter to the floor as I look for my car keys. They're not here. I hung them there this morning.

Then I understand.

He's taken them so I can't follow him. And now he knows where she's going.

49

Edie

The key sticks in Jaz's door and my heart skips. What if someone has changed the lock? I force myself to stay rational. When we found Jaz, Harry used the window, so why would they have to change the lock? My mind is racing; the smear of blood he'd left on the window frame has been wiped away. Did he mention that to the police? Increasingly agitated, I wiggle the key, twisting it, and the door swings open. The thought of Jaz lying in the front room is still with me. They would have carried her body out past where I'm standing. An unwanted image of a body bag and mortuary van waiting outside fixes itself in my mind.

Jaz's flat is in a square, overlooked by several others. I don't want curtains twitching any more than they already have been, so I gather my courage and go inside. The spare bedroom is off the front room, so I have no choice but to go through it. The rug is bare now where Jaz's body was, but otherwise the room is the same as when we left. Nothing in there moves, not even the clock on the wall. The batteries must be dead. Everything is silent as I hurry through, not wanting to spend a second longer in the flat than I have to. My clothes are where I left them in the cupboard of the spare room. I grab my charger from the desk and plug my phone in; the battery had died halfway here. While the phone is building up a few per cent of charge, I throw some things into my holdall. Just enough to escape for a few days. Clothes, toothbrush, toiletries. I don't know how long we're going to be away for. Why am I saying we? For all I know, I'm on my own. I don't even know if Harry has got my message yet.

I drop the holdall on the floor and sit on the bed, willing my phone to charge faster. I try to look anywhere but past the bedroom door to where Jaz lay. I can't believe she sank so far into despair. That was the old Jaz. The Jaz I knew might be upset initially but would then get angry and fight back. Even though she must have felt bad enough to go to the doctor and get prescribed sedatives, it's hard to imagine her taking them all. Maybe there were things I should have noticed earlier; I should have been more of a friend. But I didn't know it would come to this. Perhaps all her optimism at work was just a front, and she was hiding her real feelings from me? I put my head in my hands and close my eyes. I let the tension drain from me until the silence in the flat is humming in my ears.

After a few quiet minutes, I pick up my phone and turn it on, leaving it connected to the power. As soon as it boots up it buzzes and pings wildly. Five missed calls, all Harry.

I switch to voicemail. He is breathless.

Edie, listen, my dad has been here, he tricked me. I think he got the message you left for me. He might be on his way, so don't go to Jaz's.

There is a pause. Then message two.

Edie, please phone me when you get this. I'm worried. He's looking for you. You need to be careful. If you get this, phone me.

Pause.

Message three.

Edie? Phone me.

Pause.

Message four.

But I don't hear message four.

A hand has snaked past my shoulder and grabbed the phone from the table, tugging it roughly from the charger. I turn, but it is too late. James Creighton has grabbed my arm, and I am pulled towards him. I throw myself backwards, but it is surprising how strong he is for an older man.

'Hello, Edie.' He spits my name out as if it is a bad taste on his tongue. As I pull away, he grips me even tighter. 'Let's go. It's over.'

50

Harry

My search for the spare key is frantic. Cups roll from the cupboard, breaking on the floor. Saucepans clatter. Where the fuck is it? Tea towels, kitchen items, cutlery, all thrown and dropped. As my temper builds, the sound of breaking crockery starts to feel cathartic. The knowledge I'm not in control of what might happen next is maddening. I hate this feeling. The kitchen is an unholy mess when I finally discover the key at the back of the random item drawer, where everything we never found a proper place for ended up. I grab it; a single, black Audi key, so buried under dead batteries and old phone chargers, I'm surprised I found it at all. My father thinks of everything; I have to hand it to him; taking my keys was a stroke of genius, and I've lost fifteen minutes in the race to get to Jaz's first. Does he know where Jaz lives, though? I'm certain he'll have found out somehow. I snatch the spare house keys, lock up and run to the car.

As the engine fires, I dial my parents' house, putting my phone on speaker. I swing out into the road, heading for Jaz's flat. It's at least twenty minutes away, assuming the roads are clear. I glance at the dashboard clock. Two fifteen, I'm going to miss rush hour and I try to remember if the schools are on holiday. If so, the traffic should be okay, but then it will be okay for him as well.

Someone picks up. 'Hello?'

'Mum?'

'Harry? You sound in a hurry.'

'I am,' I tell her, heading off any small talk. 'Do you know where Dad is?'

'I think he came over to see you, Harry. He said his conference was cancelled.'

'Has he said anything to you?'

The stony silence makes me wonder if I've lost the signal. Then she speaks again. 'No, why?'

'Mum, you're lying.'

She sounds hurt. 'Look, I don't think he's up to anything, Harry. If he is, it will be for your benefit.'

'I'm glad you're so sure. Did he ever ask you about Jaz, Edie's friend? Do you remember I told you she had moved in with her after we split up?'

Again, a silence. 'Yes, he knows about her. We do share information, Harry. We're husband and wife.'

'Does he know where she lives?'

'Probably. I've always told him everything you tell me. Why shouldn't I? I wish you two would put your differences aside.'

Put our differences aside? I'm in awe of her ability to turn the other cheek wherever my father is concerned. Can you put aside the way he has stolen your personality for so many years, Mum? Or ignore the way he turned you into what he wanted you to be?

'I've got to go. I'm driving.'

I'm about to end the call when her voice crackles from the speaker again. Plaintive, lost. 'Be careful, Harry. I love you lots, you know.'

'Yeah, I know. You too, Mum.' An immense wave of pity washes over me. She is as trapped as a woman can be. She has got everything and yet nothing at all. All the houses, money, kitchens, parties and charity dinners in the world don't make up for losing yourself like she has.

I end the call as I hit slow traffic near Five Ways. I let a guttural roar of frustration out at the windscreen. Edie's phone rings out to voicemail again. On an impulse, I open Find My, and her icon pings onto the map. Her phone is back on again. How? She is still at Jaz's. As the traffic crawls, I stare at the screen. Then, without warning, the icon disappears again. Fuck.

If he gets to you Edie, fight back. You can get the better of him, I know you can. Find a way, somehow.

Once I'm past the traffic I put my foot down. I don't even consider calling the police. What would I say to them? *Oh hello, yes, I'd like to you to attend Abbotts Court because I think my father is about to section my fiancé.* I can hear the sceptical silence at the other end already. Then I could give them the *coup de grâce*, the crank call to end all crank calls. *Yes, he's the Chair of the Royal College of Psychiatrists.*

What if I'm racing there for nothing? They could just be talking. They could be ironing out their differences, realising what a big mistake it's all been. What a shock that would be; I turn up and find them having a cup of tea, best of friends. My father has nothing to hide. Edie is the perfect fiancée. Get married with my blessing, son, he says and smiles.

Yeah, right.

I know the system well enough by now. I know what she is terrified of. If he decides to section Edie, he can do it. It is supposed to take two clinicians or the police to get her in, but if he gets her to Claydon Manor he will find a way. Once she's there, it's over. She's sectioned. And then it will take two doctors to get her out. She can't just declare she is ready to leave. I've known patients kept in locked rehabilitation wards for twenty years. Begging to be released for two decades. People don't want to believe this happens in the twenty-first century, but, if a psychiatrist wants to keep someone under lock and key indefinitely, they can. The number of institutionalised patients who don't need to be there is shocking. But years down the line and there they still are. I could fight her case, get lawyers involved, but, if my father wants her locked up, then that's what will happen.

And what then? Who listens to her? If Edie and Jenny point the finger at my father, what will happen? To the whole psychiatric profession, their diagnosis will be beyond doubt. They will be seen as living in a fantasy world, conspiracy theory material; that paranoid delusion territory where people roll their eyes. Patients accusing their doctors of all sorts of crimes, harbouring grudges that turn violent, seeing lies and deception everywhere. She knows this, and

I'm praying it's enough for her to do what she needs to get away. For all of my rationalising, my logic, my pragmatism, I've known for a while what my father wants.

But he has no idea what *I* want, not yet.

I'm five minutes away from Jaz's. As I drive, I put my phone on my knee and call Edie again.

Nothing.

51

Edie

'What are you doing?' I pull free from him, but he pushes the door closed.

His face is twisted into a spiteful grimace, so different from his usual urbane and unruffled manner. His eyes travel to the bag on the floor. He shifts position, standing with his back to the closed door, blocking my exit, my phone clutched in his hand. It lights up, the upbeat ringtone jarring in the tension of the room. As he glances down, his sneer twists into a bitter smile. He shakes his head.

'Harry. My poor confused boy. You really managed to turn him against me, didn't you? Yet with everything he knows about you, he's still on your side somehow.'

I grab for the phone, but he pushes me down on the bed, his hand on my chest. His weight is on me, holding me as the phone rings out. He eases the pressure and I manage to push his hand away.

'Don't touch me.' I push myself upright. 'You did a pretty good job of turning Harry against you yourself.'

His eyes flash. 'You lying little bitch. I always did what was best for him, and he knows it. Look where he is today. With my influence, he can have whatever career he wants. He can do what he wants, and you are not going to destroy us.'

'Why would I destroy you?'

'Because it's in your nature.' He is breathing hard, almost panting. 'Because it's who you are.'

'You're crazy.' I'm laughing at him now, and his face contorts with anger. 'What's the correct term to describe what you suffer from, Professor Creighton? Psychopathy? Narcissistic Personality Disorder?

Empathy deficit? Whatever way you want to put it, it still amounts to the same thing. You're fucking insane.'

Then he hits me. The air pressure in my ear shifts as his palm arcs towards me, whipping out in a lightning movement. I don't have time to duck or turn my face. I take the blow on my temple and then I'm on the bed in a foetal position, my vision exploding with bursts of white light. The bedroom shimmers and swims before juddering back into focus. Creighton is standing over me, baring his teeth in animal rage. Whatever Harry said about his father, he was only touching the surface. Harry's hatred doesn't go deep enough. Now I see the man who would have belittled him all his life, ruling by ridicule, shame. Guilt. A man whose hair-trigger temper meant violence was never far away. When Harry told me his father was never physically violent, I know now, he was lying. Boys are ashamed when they're bullied, so how must it feel as a man? As the sting of the slap lingers on the side of my cheek, I understand when the seeds of shame are planted. In childhood.

But so are the seeds of defiance. So is the ability to fight back.

Creighton is bending over me. 'You don't get to say that to me. Not after what you've done. Do you hear?'

Before I can overthink it, my left foot lashes out and connects solidly with his shin.

His shriek of pain is high and shrill as he drops my phone. I gather it from the floor and then I'm running. I half-spin as my shoulder slams against the doorjamb, then I'm out into the hall, his footsteps behind me.

'Come back.' His voice is ragged, a few feet behind me. Ahead, the front door is now closed, although I'd left it ajar. I try to take it in one movement, opening it, running through, then closing it. But I stumble and the door catches my foot. It flies open again and Creighton is behind me, two metres, one metre. He is slim and fit. Athletic.

I turn and swing, the phone in my hand catching him a lucky blow on his cheek. The case cracks against bone and he staggers back as the phone flies from my hand, looping and arcing, landing heavily in the parking lot. It shatters, small fragments flying in the air and skittering across the concrete, catching the afternoon sun, which has broken through the clouds. I stumble towards my car, dimly aware of someone watching, distant. Then I'm against the car door, and Creighton is on me. He uses all his weight to push against me, grabbing my wrists.

'You've done all the damage you're going to do,' he hisses. His fingers are searching, grasping, trying to control my hands as I twist and turn, my feet skidding and scraping against the floor, scrabbling for purchase. We are face to face, inches apart. I can smell his breath, see the pure rage in his eyes. His hair has flopped across his forehead, and his hand is reaching for my throat. 'Get in the car. Don't make this difficult.'

Who is the passer-by watching us? Why aren't they helping? I can just make her out: an elderly neighbour who has come out of her flat with a small dog on a lead. She's stopped, staring across to the car. The pale blob of her face is at the edge of my vision. Why is she just staring?

I try to call to her, but my voice is lost in the struggle.

I twist one more time, my shoulder screaming in protest as I bend double and rip it free. Then I'm away, running along the narrow road.

There is no way to get off the road, and I hear his car start behind me. The engine noise increases as he closes on me. My head swivels, left, right, but there is no way out. I can hear his car catching up with me and I'm fifty yards from the main road.

In seconds the engine noise of the car is behind me, revving hard. I think of Harry and wonder if his family are as capable of murder as mine. I keep running, and, as the car approaches, I know they are. As I glance back, I stumble and fall again, and this time I don't have the strength to back get up.

The engine noise gets closer and I wait for the impact.

52

Harry

I pull into Jaz's street and race to the bottom of the road where the flats are, getting some dirty looks from pedestrians trying to cross at the junction. Edie's car is parked in one of the bays, but there's no sign of my father's. Her car is locked, so I run across the parking area and to the front door. It's ajar; my throat tightens. I push it all the way open. 'Anyone there?' Silence.

The front room is empty, and the door to the spare bedroom is open. Edie's bag, almost fully packed, is spilled on the floor. An iPhone charging wire hangs from a plug, which is half-pulled from the wall.

I already know there's no one here, but I shout anyway. 'Edie?'

I go through the routine of checking the cupboards and under the bed, as if she's playing hide and seek. What if he got here while she was packing? If her car is here and she's not, it must mean she has either escaped or he has got her. Outside, I skirt around the flat. Nothing. Her number goes straight to voicemail. I try my father's number with the same result. Find My is empty.

Then I spot the debris in the corner of the parking lot and finally understand. Glass, plastic and electronic components litter the concrete. There is a half-intact phone case, some screen fragments. It's hers, I recognise the cover immediately.

As I stare listlessly at the broken phone pieces, a voice interrupts my thoughts.

'Are you looking for the young lady?' The woman speaking is in her seventies. At her feet, a small dog on a tartan lead bounces up at me, barking. 'Shush now, Milo,' the woman whispers, and the dog falls silent, watching me with suspicious brown eyes.

'Yes. Did you see what happened?' I ask.

She nods. 'Well, there was bit of an argument here. She ran off.'

'Who was she arguing with?'

'An older man, in his fifties. To be honest, from where I was standing, I thought it was a father and daughter having a row. He was very aggressive, but it was only when he drove off after her I realised how serious the situation was. I'm sorry, I didn't know what to do.'

'Have you phoned the police?'

'No, not yet. I wasn't sure whether I should?'

Even if I tried to explain, I doubt she'd understand how the police would immediately take his side once they learned it was a clinical matter. A mental health issue. And that's exactly how my father would frame it. If they did get involved, it would be to help him, not her.

'No, it's too late now,' I tell her. 'It's a… family dispute. Which way did they go?'

'She ran off that way, and he chased her in the car.'

'How long ago?'

'Only about five minutes.'

I run towards my car. Her voice follows me. 'What should I do?'

But I'm already in the car and pulling away. If he's planning to section her, there is only one place he will be going. I can't help her any more. All I can do is hope she can get away from him. That she will do what I hope she is capable of.

Because if he gets her in there, she won't be coming out again.

53

Edie

I don't feel any impact, just the skid of tyres as he stops next to me. My breath is coming in short, ragged bursts, and I have no fight left. He pulls me from where I've fallen and into the passenger side of the car, locking me in, then opens the driver's side manually with the key. He is driving away in less than thirty seconds. In the middle of the day, a woman has been abducted, and nobody has done a thing. Then we are out onto the Hagley Road and into the traffic. For several moments, neither of us speaks. He pushes his hair back from his brow and smooths it down, regaining his composure.

'You shouldn't have fought me,' he says eventually. 'I'm not in the habit of striking women, but I had no choice.' No choice. So it was my fault, was it? I try the door handle, but he is already picking up speed as he clears the traffic. He notices and smiles. 'Don't bother, it's on lock.'

Outside, a sunlit park rolls by. Dog walkers and joggers circulate, oblivious. I don't need to gauge the direction we're going in, I already know. Claydon Manor. I turn to Creighton with a sneer. 'No, you don't hit women. Unless they do something you don't like.'

He shakes his head, now back to his calm, rational self. Back to the James Creighton I've come to know over the last two years. 'Not true, I'm afraid. Much as you'd probably like it to be.'

'Where are you taking me?' Engaging him in conversation might give me time to think.

'Isn't it obvious?' He takes a long look in the rear-view mirror as if checking we're not being followed. 'You need help, you know you do. You need protecting from yourself.'

279

I snort. 'So says the man who punched me in the head?'

'As I said, you don't get to question my actions. Not where my family are concerned.'

'And what about my family? What about my mother? You don't care how much you hurt *us*, do you?'

A loud bray of incredulous laughter comes from him. 'The only people who have ever hurt you and Jenny Carter—' he looks directly at me for a moment '—are you and Jenny Carter.'

A deep sense of injustice drags at my gut, as though things have been unfair from the moment I was born. As if there is no point in fighting against a destiny that seems to follow me everywhere. But then I haven't yet reached a stage in my life where I've given up. I've always fought for what I know to be right. And it's this sense of fight that won't let me accept the status quo. It fuels the burning hatred that makes me determined for this man – this powerful, arrogant man – not to get away with it this time. Makes me desperate to show him that I know what his real motives are.

'I'm starting to remember what happened, and that's bothering you, isn't it?'

He doesn't let me unnerve him. He is calm, in control. 'It should be bothering you more than me. I have nothing to hide.'

'Given your unethical treatment of my mother, you have everything to hide. And you have more to lose than I do.'

'In that particular statement, you might be right.'

'You're going to section me, aren't you? You want to keep me under observation.'

He smiles, self-assured. Secure in his authority and enjoying every moment of it. 'Yes, of course. When we get to the centre, I'm going to admit you for assessment. If you resist, or try to run, or get angry, or do any of those things I know you're desperate to do, we will put you under a Section Two. This will give us twenty-eight days to get something more permanent in place.'

'And Morris is on your side, isn't he?'

'Doctor Morris has always been very supportive of my requests. But he doesn't know about your admission to the unit yet. He doesn't know I've come to find you, or the extent of…' Creighton has the nerve to pause for a moment. 'He doesn't understand the extent of your mental issues. I purposely kept him in the dark about most things. The same goes for Amy Wilson. I don't want my family name dragged through the mud.'

We're now driving through the Warwickshire countryside. We are going too fast for me to jump out, even if I could open the door. Creighton has achieved a *fait accompli*; when we get to the centre, any resistance from me will look like either paranoia or a tendency towards violence, which will prove his point. The only option I have is to keep him talking.

'Why are you doing this? Jenny's husband was an abuser. Michael Carter. My so-called father.'

'Michael Carter may or may not have been an abuser. Who knows? That's hardly the point. He's long dead.'

'It's precisely the fucking point for me,' I explode, my voice deafening in the confined space of the car. 'My mother and I have buried this for years, you arrogant bastard. Half of my life is missing.'

'Oh, you've buried your past, have you? From whom, may I ask?' His smile has taken on the predatory smirk I've associated with him ever since we met. 'I'm protective of my family, young lady. I'm aware of the attack at Claydon Manor. I know that violence is never far away where you and Jenny are concerned. You forget I am just as capable of investigating the past as you are.'

'What's that supposed to mean?' Anger is rising; so is panic. The seatbelt feels too tight across my chest, as if it is strangling me. My breathing comes in short, rapid bursts, as my voice takes on an edge of hysteria. 'What are you trying to say?'

'Jenny is surprisingly talkative when she is interviewed in the right way. She talked about the abduction long before I ever got to Claydon Manor. It was all in her notes.'

'So that's how Richard Morris and Amy Wilson knew who Samuel Cox was before I did? It came from you.'

'Yes, with some help from Jenny. And with the right type of medication, of course.'

'That's illegal. Unethical.'

'Oh please. Stop pretending you care about her.' He has the condescending tone of someone talking to a troublesome child. 'Jenny Carter hates you, you know.'

We are cresting the brow of a hill, and the green, rolling landscape draws me in, relieving the claustrophobia of the car. As Creighton's words sink into my consciousness, I don't have any more answers. All I can do is stare across the broad, scenic valley that is opening up in front of me. Why is the world so unfair? Everything consists of beauty and misery in equal measure, and we don't always get to choose which one our lives are made of. While some people get it all, others get nothing. A wave of sadness engulfs me because I know Creighton is right. My mother does hate me. She hates me and she blames me. The guilt is both of ours to share. Perhaps talking to Creighton, getting it all out, was a relief for her. But that admission is for me and me alone. I wouldn't give him the satisfaction of telling him.

'She doesn't hate me,' I protest. My voice is quiet, uncertain. I'm not even convincing myself. 'We love each other.'

Creighton's crafty smile widens. 'She might have loved you once. She might even have felt sorry for you. But she never loved you the way she loved Edie.'

'*I* am Edie.'

I feel like crying. My voice is scared and hesitant, the same as that young girl I used to be all those years ago. The young girl who played on the beach, who envied the lives of the family that took her in each day, and who cried herself to sleep in the bitter, austere room of her care home.

His eyes are hard, unforgiving. 'Edie's dead, isn't she? And you know how it happened.'

The statement is simple and clear. He shatters my world in a tone of voice so flat, so emotionless, he may as well have been discussing the weather. All those things my mother said recently as she held me so close are flooding back. That afternoon in her room when she told me who I really am, tore down all those years of dissociation and denial. We are on a straight piece of road, and Creighton twists again to look me straight in the eye. In his gaze is everything I've known since my mother whispered the truth into my ear. He has been doing all of this to protect his son; he is doing it to protect his family.

After all, who would want their son engaged to someone like me?

'Edie's dead,' he repeats, as calmly as ever. 'Isn't she, Sophie?'

The only noise is the hum of the tyres on the road, and the rush of air as cars pass us in the opposite direction.

Can Edie really be dead? It's as though I'm remembering someone I met once, a long time ago. Someone I loved. And I did truly love her; everyone must believe that, they have to.

My mother must believe it.

And she *is* my mother; just because she didn't give birth to me doesn't mean she doesn't love me like the daughter she lost.

She loves me just as much as she loved Edie.

Edie.

More beautiful than me, more gifted. More troubled. I loved her, I hated her. I wanted to *be* her. I wanted what she had, what I could never get. All those years, with just one week in the summer together. I can still see the colour of the dinghy we used to play in the sea with. We used to paddle out so far, until the shore was a shimmering green line in the distance. The sun was high, glinting off the water. We would float there, lying on our backs, letting the dinghy drift, with no knowledge of tides and currents. She would lean out and dip her hand in the water as she watched the sun sparkle and play, letting her fingers sway on the surface with the lapping of the sea, back and forth. I can see her long hair, just like mine. I wore it like she did. Everyone said we could be sisters. When I heard that, the thrill of thinking my life could be like hers would bubble up in me. It would fill my heart with hope. But it could never quite fill the void.

Thick, hot tears burn my cheeks. I am crying now in front of him. It's as if he can see the memories in my mind as I weep, watching them like a film. He can read them all, he can read what really happened, and everything I am is open to him. Every lie, every deceit. Every stolen memory, lost in the recesses of my mind. He knows who I am, what I did.

And so do I.

Then, Creighton is talking. Twisting the truth into me like a jagged, rusty knife.

'I knew straight away your memory loss wasn't consistent with traumatic dissociation. Even if Amy Wilson couldn't see that, I could. I'm certain that you truly believed your own lies, but I came to understand that Jenny, Edie's mother, held all of the secrets of the past, which you didn't want to come to light. She has been carrying guilt all her life. She was already traumatised about letting Edie be abused by Michael. I know what she did to her husband; I know she killed him. Once I had got past her denial, she couldn't wait to admit it to me. She... how can I put it? *Facilitated* his suicide when he was drunk. She was even proud of it, I think. But it will have to be reported to the police now, of course. Regardless of what Michael did to Edie, it is still murder.'

'You don't understand. She *wanted* me to be Edie.'

'No, she didn't. You manipulated her, Sophie.'

Doesn't he see? Doesn't he understand? 'No, you weren't there. She wanted me to be her. When Edie...' I stop, unable to say the word. How do I explain the pain of watching her drown? 'When Edie died...'

'Edie drowning wasn't an accident though, Sophie, was it?'

'She couldn't swim well,' I shout. 'She fell in. I couldn't help her, we were too far out. When she didn't come home, Jenny wanted me to be her daughter. She wanted me to be Edie. She needed a chance to make it up to her. I was all she had left.'

He smiles, that horrible, knowing grin. That institutional smile, the one I know so well. 'Jenny hates you, and you know it. She still pretends you're Edie, but she won't even look at you when she says her name, will she?'

'That's not true.'

'You killed Edie that day on the dinghy, didn't you? You pushed her off and watched her drown.'

'No. If I did that, why would Jenny look after me?'

'Sophie, like all pathological liars, you managed to persuade her. She was already vulnerable, wracked with remorse. It was you who preyed on her weakness. It was you who preyed on her guilt. She was ready to be manipulated.'

'No, she wanted it.'

He will never understand how Jenny wanted it this way. She begged me to be Edie, she wanted to give me the love that Edie had. I was as close to her as a daughter. Why should I give up the chance of a family?

He shakes his head, so sure of himself. 'Your lies are falling apart. You reported yourself as missing, instead of Edie. You persuaded Jenny not to turn you in, to maintain the lie. There was a search, and police made enquiries. But the search soon tailed off. Sophie was troubled; she had a history of running away. She had no family. Multiple failed foster placements. Jenny was already in the throes of a nervous breakdown because of the abuse. You manipulated her, and once the lie was accepted there was no going back. You're a cuckoo, Sophie. You took Edie's place.'

'No, it wasn't like that. You've got it wrong.'

'I know Jenny told you the truth that day with Stefan. She told me all about it afterwards. I do believe your selective repression was genuine until then, but that moment destroyed it. From then on, your investigations were just a way of finding out what people actually remembered about you. To see whether the deception would hold. Your visits to your mother were to find out what she had already told me. You were interrogating her like you thought I would. You just wanted to know if she would break.'

'You're lying.'

The sun slants through the window, touching my face. It feels good. I don't want to hear any more, but he keeps talking, relentless. 'In the four years since the abduction, before you watched her drown, Edie told you everything. She told you about the abuse, she told you about being taken, all the details of what happened. She told you about the cottage, how it looked, how it felt. She told you her that her father

285

was dead, even how her mother broke the news to her. You took on all of these memories as your own, and then proceeded to bury the ones that reminded you of who you were. In the following years, you have developed a quite impressive dissociative personality. Denial is an incredibly powerful thing, Sophie.'

'I'm Edie.' My voice is weaker than ever, like a whisper coming from the past, a memory fading into nothingness. I'm so quiet now he doesn't hear me.

'Jenny allowed the deception to be internalised. It's called transference; you became Edie and, with your help, she convinced herself you were her missing daughter. Who would ever know? You looked similar, and she moved towns and schools that summer. Neither Michael nor Jenny had any close family to ask questions. It was just the two of you. Finally, in her mind, you became Edie. But the lie never really took for her.' His voice hardens. 'And the truth comes out in other ways.'

'That's a lie. Samuel Cox was my father. I cried when he died.'

'You cried for yourself, not him. Samuel Cox was Edie's biological father. He was about to wake up and, the moment he saw you, he would know you weren't the real Edie. I don't know who you manipulated to get your job back, but after that he was at your mercy, and you managed to make sure he never did wake up to see you.'

'No. Jaz made the drug error.'

'Jaz was innocent, wasn't she?'

Was she? I think back to the drugs cupboard. The drugs check. The metronidazole was in a plastic vial. It wasn't difficult for me to inject the fentanyl into it while she was distracted. I'd already drawn it up in theatres, left the syringe in my scrubs. Samuel Cox was the only patient in the unit who was on metronidazole. It would have to be administered to him. I stare at Creighton, my mind full of molten rage.

What does he know about me? How dare he judge what I did? Okay, you smug bastard. Maybe it would be easier if Sam was dead. Jaz didn't know I'd spiked the metronidazole. But it could have been Matt who gave it, it could have been anyone. I was sorry it was Jaz who gave it, don't you see that? I *liked* her, for fuck's sake.

'Do you know what it's like to be born with nothing?' I shout. 'To be brought up in a dozen different houses. To be kicked from pillar to post, with no one who truly gives a fuck about you. You'd love me to be that cliché; the care home kid's always the villain, right?'

'That doesn't come into it.'

'You have everything, so how could you know me?' I stare down at my thumb where blood is running from the nail. That stress habit I've had ever since I was little. I remember it bleeding that day at the beach, and Sam dressing it for me. I'd lied about cutting it on a rock. I did love him, despite what this man thinks. 'Can't you see how much I needed what Edie had? A future? A mother who loved her?'

'So you just stole her identity?' I realise I'm just another case to him. I just happen to be engaged to his son. Somehow, I understand it's not personal any more. He takes his eyes from the road long enough to meet my blurred, teary eyes. 'Well, it's all over now, Sophie.'

We'll be at Claydon Manor in a few minutes. He turns back to the road and there's no more time to think as we crest the ridge of the hill. The click of his seatbelt latch as I press the red button and release it is loud enough for him to look down. He frowns, his grey eyes losing all of their arrogance, their entitlement, their certainty, as he realises what I've done. His seatbelt slides across him and back into its holder as I pull mine to make sure it's in place. I have enough time to glance at the speedometer before I grab the wheel.

Sixty-five. A steep incline.

Traumatic injury and collision scenarios rush through my mind in milliseconds; mechanism of injury, speed of impact, possibility of survival. My seatbelt is secure, his isn't. I give him a twenty-five per cent chance. If the car flips over, fifteen. I give myself sixty.

'What are you doing?' he cries. He is caught between wrestling the wheel back and fastening his seatbelt again. In the end, he does neither. 'Sophie. No.'

But the sound of his last words is lost in the screech of tyres on tarmac, as I pull the wheel hard to the left and the car slews towards the lip of the road. The front wheel clips a tree root, and I brace myself against the door frame as the car tips, and we're rolling, pitching and sliding down the embankment towards a small copse of trees, crashing and screeching towards a sea of solid trunks.

Then there is noise, the smash of the windscreen, deafening sounds of crimping metal and cracking timber. Steam hissing from the engine, metal shearing.

And finally, silence.

My vision fades for a moment, but I force myself to stay awake. I keep still for several seconds, mentally assessing myself for injuries. I move my arms and legs, check for blood.

Pain shoots through my shoulder. I feel it; it's not dislocated.

The driver's seat is now empty; Creighton has been thrown through the windscreen. He is lying five metres away, twisted against a tree, not moving, his blood-matted hair plastered across his face. Dimly aware of cars stopping at the top of the ridge, out of the line of sight, I pull myself free of the wreckage.

Then I am clear and running. Along a hedgerow, past a field, toward a nearby village.

I'm not Sophie Cullen. Sophie drowned many years ago. I worked hard to get where I am. I deserve this life.

I'm Doctor Edie Carter. Sophie is dead.

That's what James Creighton couldn't understand.

54

Sophie

It's been two weeks since the crash, but the pain still lingers as I sit up in bed when my old alarm clock buzzes.

'Why don't you call in sick? Come back to bed.' Harry's suggestion is beyond tempting. He tries again, his hand on my back. 'Come on, Edes. Your shoulder is still sore, remember?'

'Harry, I'm going to be late for work, and so are you.'

He sits up and throws a leg either side of me, so we are spooning in a sitting position.

He rests his head on my shoulder and kisses it.

'Yeah, but I feel kind of responsible.'

'Why?'

He pushes closer, his lips on my cheek. 'Why do you think?'

'Forget it,' I say. 'How are you feeling?'

'I can't quite believe it of him. No one can. How did he lose it like that? But Jaz's neighbour said he was being aggressive. I'm glad you managed to get away from him at the flats. He must have been in such a rage to grab you hard enough to injure your shoulder, and drive away like he did.'

'Look, I don't want to do a hatchet job on him, Harry, considering what happened afterwards.'

'Yeah, I know.' Harry rubs my neck. 'But I'm not blind to what his temper was like; I was brought up by him, remember?' He kisses my shoulder again, and his arms snake around my waist. His chest and stomach are warm against me.

'I'm sorry about what happened to him,' I said. 'Truly sorry.'

'I know, but it wasn't your fault.'

'I just feel bad accusing him now. I don't suppose it matters any more, does it?'

'I love you, Edie,' he whispers into the curve of my ear. The feel of his breath sends a pleasant ripple down my back.

'I know,' I reply, then wriggle free and stand up, turning to face him. I kiss him, resisting the urge to turn the kiss into something more. 'But that doesn't change the fact I'm going to be late.'

I shower quickly, thinking about Morris. He has been surprisingly nice to me in recent days, and was very understanding about my taking a few days off work for my shoulder and neck. It's easy to pull the trapezius muscle, he'd said, and very painful. Harry had wanted what happened between me and his father at Jaz's kept quiet, understandably. After all, there were still reputations to be considered, and I didn't want Harry's being tarnished because his father had a vendetta against me. It was easy enough to claim I'd fought Creighton off after he'd chased me in the car, driving like a madman. And who could disprove that I'd given him the slip and made my way home? Why tell anyone about the things he had accused my mother and me of? As far as anyone was concerned, he was driving on his own when he lost control on the brow of a hill and rolled down the embankment.

My mother was pleased that he wouldn't be her consultant any longer; she was as upset as I was about the way he had handled us both. It was just lucky he hadn't made his suspicions public yet, and he had kept his ridiculous assumptions to himself. Morris was as devastated as anyone about the crash, particularly as James Creighton had always taken such an interest in my welfare. He asked me to pass his condolences to Harry. Morris was even more pleased when I agreed to take up my sessions with Amy Wilson again. I was sorry I'd been fighting her, I told him, I should accept that resistance makes things worse. The sooner I come to terms with the terrible things that had happened to me in the past, the easier I would find it. He admitted he could have been more understanding, telling me he realised my statements about Cox's innocence were through shock, and of course I would want to be involved in patient care. He hoped

I understood why he wanted to protect me, though. I'd nodded and smiled.

Of course, Doctor Morris.

Our relationship has become more harmonious now, and Morris has told me that when he signs me off next month my references will be excellent. I've always wanted to work in a large London teaching hospital, where I can apply for specialist training, and pass my skills on to other up-and-coming anaesthetists, so that's probably what I'll aim for. Maybe St Thomas' or UCH, as it had always been the dream. Somewhere I can get ahead and climb the ladder.

Harry is dressed when I get back into the bedroom. Everyone at his work has been sympathetic as well, and they have given him time off as he needs it. He has decided to go in today; it's better to keep busy. I towel-dry my hair and pull my jeans and a hoodie on.

'Hey, Edes. Don't forget about tonight,' he says.

Tonight? Oh yes, of course. Dinner with his mother. 'Yeah, okay. I'll be home about six.'

'Great. It'll just be us. She needs the company, you know. I don't think she likes being alone right now.'

'No Nicky this time then?'

He grins, shakes his head. 'Boy, you really hold a grudge, don't you? No, no Nicky, right? No more Nicky ever, just you and me.'

'You think?'

'I know, Edie.' He holds my hand and gives me that look. We kiss again, slowly. 'It's always been you.'

It has been nearly three weeks since Jaz died, but the shock is still palpable at the morning huddle at the nurses' station. The funeral had been the previous week and Matt had been inconsolable. He took several days leave, and when he came back he looked awful, as though he hadn't been sleeping. As Jaz's best friend, I've been the one to take him for coffees, talk to him, and do my best to convince him there is nothing he could have done. But he is still beating himself up; I should have been there for her, he repeats whenever we talk about it, but I think gradually he is beginning to understand that no one could have foreseen how hard the suspension would hit her, me included.

The morning huddle gets done in a perfunctory *let's get through this* sort of way. There are no new patients overnight, nothing to make me think the shift is going to be anything other than what I had hoped for, as I ease myself back into the rigours of Intensive Care. Jaz has been replaced by a humourless temporary nurse called Maureen, who is constantly obsessed by how much extra money she gets through doing agency work. It doesn't go down too well with the rest of the team; some of the other nurses are extremely pissed off that someone doing the same job as them is earning much more than they are, and when the morning meeting breaks up I have to lift their spirits as it's what Jaz would have wanted. Although Jaz is irreplaceable, the interviews for someone to fill her role are now in progress. In a month or two, Maureen will be sent somewhere else.

Morris is not in today, so we have Victoria Armitage as our consultant. She is nice enough, but ineffective in emergency situations. In her late forties, dripping in bangles and rings despite the 'bare below the elbows' regime that is supposed to be strictly adhered to in theatres and ICU, she swans around the department, overseeing things but doing very little work herself. More often than not, the actual work is left to the juniors, and the newly trained medics. Doctors much like me, in fact. Doctor Armitage's chief concern seems to be how her horses are doing, and when she will next have time to ride them. It's not as if she has to work, anyway. Her husband is a consultant plastic surgeon who does one NHS list a week, and then makes an eye-watering fortune practising privately.

That kind of life will never be for me; give me the cut-and-thrust of front-line medicine any day. I want to be where life and death are balanced precariously; I want to be the one making the difference, pulling people through, fighting to keep people alive. Everyone deserves a chance to live, and that's why emergency and intensive care medicine is so addictive and thrilling. In those minutes, you make the difference. What you do counts, and how you react defines whether people live or die. It's power, yes, but it's also responsibility.

I know medical ethics inside out; some people claim certain patients don't deserve the same chances others do, for example. I don't agree. Everyone should be treated equally. Of course, that is a slight generalisation. I'm not sure it applies to people who have wronged me personally. I think I'd feel differently about whether they deserved a chance then.

I sit at the desk as the morning huddle breaks up and the staff go about their business.

People disappear into various areas and the unit is quiet once more, apart from the familiar hiss of ventilators and the occasional ping of monitors. I am at home in here. Across the empty department is Samuel Cox's bay, the place where he lay for so many days, hovering between life and death. It was a shame he didn't pull through. Well, at least for some people. He wasn't a bad man. Maybe he deserved better. But we doctors aren't gods. I pull my mask up to cover my mouth and nose. It is one of those protocols that sometimes gets forgotten. People tend to just wear them around their necks or across their mouth. Wearing the mask properly covers the whole of the lower face; sometimes it can even make your own colleagues unrecognisable.

I stroll towards Cox's old bay, remembering everything that went on there. My memory is better now; it is still selective when I talk to Amy Wilson and Richard Morris. They don't need to know everything. Maybe I was a little paranoid before; they were doing what they thought was best for me, after all. Most people were. But there were people who would do me harm, who were trying to hurt Jenny and me. That was a different matter and couldn't be tolerated. I look at the bay, and the person now occupying the space where Samuel Cox used to be.

How ironic.

James Creighton looks a different man to the one I used to know, as he lies unconscious. His hair is short now, and bald in clumps where his head was shaved for the neurosurgery that saved his life. But although they stabilised him, the long-term neurological damage looks less promising. Morris weaned him off the ventilator after ten days, and now Creighton is breathing for himself. But there is no sign so far that he has regained any neurological function. His brain stem, controlling his autonomic functions – his breathing, his circulation – is intact. So far, though, no one knows how much else of his brain function has survived. There is talk of him being transferred to a specialised neurology ICU soon, perhaps in the next day or two. Maybe he will never regain consciousness.

But maybe he will.

So many unanswered questions. Perhaps he should have voiced his concerns earlier, made his accusations known before finding me. Before slapping me, insulting me. Before trying to lock me up. Maybe he should have brought the police with him. Perhaps he should have let someone else know about his suspicions before he tried to ruin my life. But he didn't. And now those things he believes about me, all those lies he told, are locked in that damaged brain.

And none of it may ever come out.

Still, better not to take any chances.

I've decided on a strong muscle relaxant; suxamethonium. It is processed by the body rapidly and has a short half-life. It leaves no trace. If I give just the right amount, it will stop him breathing long enough to make sure he never talks again. Another cardiac arrest on the ward? This time, Victoria Armitage can deal with it. I allow myself a smile beneath my mask; with her working on him, his chances are even slimmer.

I pull the curtains across, muting the alarms on the monitor so no one will come. I loosen the oxygen saturation probe on his finger just to be certain.

I deserve this chance of happiness. I know Harry loves me. Do I love him? I think so, but that doesn't mean we're forever. Perhaps I'll take off on my own somewhere after qualifying. He has shown flashes of temper. He has occasionally been a little controlling, and that is a red flag.

Harry thinks we were meant to be. Maybe he's right, but maybe not. After all, what brought us together? We were two damaged people, and we complemented each other perfectly. So we'll see.

Maybe I can see myself moving on from him eventually. I hate being tied down.

I look down at his father. Harry will be upset about this, at first. But I will help him come to terms with it.

I deserve this life. I've worked hard enough to make it mine.

The suxamethonium ampoules are still cold from where I removed them from the drug fridge. I crack them open and begin drawing up.

Part of a doctor's role is to know when to help people. James Creighton may well be in a vegetative state.

I look upon this as an act of mercy.

Epilogue
Harry

She leaves for work, and I sit down with a coffee. I have half an hour before I need to go myself. Enough time to reflect upon how our lives have changed in the past few weeks. It seems strange to think it was less than two months ago Samuel Cox arrived and turned everything upside down. Now he is gone, and Jaz is gone, and my mother is in that large house on her own. She will need taking care of, looking after. None of this was her fault.

She shouldn't be the one to suffer.

Edie was right when she said my father didn't like her from the beginning. She was also right that I *did* like her, right from the moment we set eyes on each other. There was something about her that struck a deep, true note somewhere in me, like two people in the same key. We have had difficult moments, of course – all couples do – but most of the time we are solid. Love doesn't even cover it; it's deeper than that, and now we have a life together, which no one can take away from us. When all of this was happening, I was always on her side. I was prepared to choose her over my own father. Surely that's saying something about commitment?

Yes, I chose her over him, despite his hold on me. I knew I would never be rid of him without extreme measures. There's something oppressive about the way some children can never be truly free while their parents are alive. Perhaps that's morbid, but for me, at least, it's true. And what happens when the relationship with one parent is so toxic the child would be prepared to go through anything to escape it?

Edie doesn't know half of it. She is fixated on her own truth, not mine. She doesn't know how much I wanted to be shot of him. It could

296

have ended so differently. I might have lost Edie instead. But somehow, I knew she would act exactly as she did, that she would find a way. I knew she would fight, because that's who she is. When I say we know each other as though we are two sides of the same person, I'm serious. I understand the lengths she will go to in order to protect herself and the life she's built. She understands how I feel too; we are kindred spirits. But on this one, I had to hide my agenda from her. Sorry, Edie. But I'll make sure I never hide who I am again in the future.

And we *do* have a future. A long and happy one.

I take a crumpled, well-read letter from my pocket, its fragments carefully taped back together. As soon as my father's letter was in the bin, those torn-up scraps of paper had nagged me, pulled at me. I was always inquisitive as a child. A quiet, sensitive, curious boy. How easily I must have broken and lost my sense of self. But how glad I am my curiosity survived, that it got the better of me, and I listened to that nagging voice and pulled those white slivers from the bin the next morning. Reattached them carefully.

In his flowing script, he had explained himself. Told me everything. I stare at his handwriting. Will I ever see him again after this? Who knows? I don't think he is going to get any better. I don't think she will give him a chance to. I smooth the letter with my palm, scan the neat lines written across it. The paper is expensive, watermarked, the writing is in fountain pen. Those touches are so like him.

His writing is old-fashioned, almost formal. Coolly and rationally, he explains what he discovered about Edie. How he'd always had his suspicions about her condition. How he has spent the weeks since Samuel Cox arrived in the ICU investigating her.

I do not have proof yet but I soon will. Edie is not who she says she is. She is hiding behind her condition. She is an impostor.

You finally got your proof, didn't you? You finally got it out of Jenny. You discovered who she really was. But you were too scared of your reputation to make it public. You wanted to keep it all under wraps, deal with it yourself.

This is why I will go to any lengths to keep you two apart.

I scan his diagnosis of her. Dissociative personality disorder with attendant psychopathy. That's a long way of saying she's fucked up. But Dad, aren't we all?

And then, the biggest insult of all, towards the end of your beautifully phrased letter.

I know I've sometimes been hard on you in the past. We all make mistakes, Harry. This is my way of repairing them.

Repairing your mistakes? You don't know what you've created. You don't know the type of man I am now. Just as I never knew you properly, just as I only knew the anger, the bitterness and the arrogance. But I soaked it all up, internalised it, as children do. We never knew each other, you and I, so why would you ever think what we have is repairable?

Oh, I knew there were things she was hiding from me. I may not have known the whole truth, but, when you told it to me in your letter, it was with a sense of sublime freedom that I discovered I didn't care. You never understood how much I love her and how blind love can be. You never realised how strongly we were united over this. There is something that holds us together. We had a shared value, which means we are the perfect match.

Our hatred of you.

Our hatred of the past, of where we come from, and of the things that happened to us. We recognise it in each other.

And I knew what she was capable of. I knew that you'd met your match in her. At Jaz's flat, I saw all the things Jaz wrote down about the day in the drug cupboard, checking drugs. Jaz began suspecting the drugs had been tampered with, and that's why she grew distant with Edie. She encouraged Jaz to write the notes to see what she remembered. Then she planned to go through them with her to make sure she wasn't incriminated, but the guilt and shame of the suspension got to Jaz first. It was a very convincing show of grief at Jaz's flat, when we found her body, though maybe Edie saw what Jaz had done to herself as one more problem solved. But Jaz's suspicions were all there in those pages I tore from the pad. I didn't want either Edie or the police finding the pages, which pointed out she had ready access to fentanyl, and that she was the one who had checked the metronidazole that was given to Cox.

And if I stoked Edie's paranoia about your intentions, Dad, I make no apologies. She mistrusted you already, so it didn't take much to add fuel to the fire, to make her believe she was going to be sectioned for life, studied, categorised. That your intentions were all bad. To prevent that, Edie would do whatever she had to, and in the end she didn't need any help from me; she did it all for herself. It just took me to mention a fictional conversation between you and Amy Wilson, supposedly overheard by Beth Lafferty. Edie was only too willing to believe that you knew we were back together, and that was all it needed for me to plant the seed that you were coming for her. That you were going to section her to get her away from me. Beth Lafferty didn't overhear the conversation because it never happened.

In the end, just planting that seed in Edie's mind, and keeping it watered, was enough to drive her to desperate measures. Then all I had to do was leave my phone unlocked the morning you told me you were coming to get her, leave the front door on the latch, play the surprised, outraged son. I knew you couldn't resist checking my messages to discover where she was, I knew you would want to do this by yourself. Avoid the scandal at all costs, don't jeopardise our reputations. And all I could do was hope that she was the one who came through it, not you. Hope that she found a way to outwit you.

And she did.

So you survived. That was a shame, but I know she will find a way to keep her secret safe, just as it will be safe with me. You were the architect of your own downfall; you underestimated her. I won't make the same mistake. You might have been fascinated by her pathology. But I know her inside out. Call it an obsession if you like.

I hold the letter for a few more moments, looking at his writing, his excuses. Too little too late. The damage is already done. The damage was done years ago.

At the stove, the click of the ignition is loud, as the gas ring bursts into life. A blue-orange flame forms, perfectly circular, hissing ferociously. I watch it for a moment, and then hold the letter to it.

The paper catches, a quick yellow tongue, running across the page, consuming the writing. Then it is gone and a blank corner remains as ash floats towards the extractor fan, the last remnants of the life of Sophie Cullen.

So now we are bound together, you and I, Sophie. I know what you've done, I know who you are. I can turn you in any time I wish. I can destroy you, just like he thought *he* could.

And you'll see what type of man I can be. I'll keep your secret, as long as you do things my way. I've kept my temper under wraps with you so far, I've really made an effort. But there's no reason to pretend anymore, and it'll be a relief to finally be myself. As long as you love me, obey me, you'll see how devoted I can be. If not, you don't want to find out how bad it can get for you. But let's not think that way. We'll have a wonderful life together.

You are mine now, Sophie. I own you.

And I don't care what you call yourself.

Because after all, what's in a name?

Acknowledgements

I would like to thank my brilliant agent Francesca for all her patience, advice, good humour, and for getting this book out there, and all at the Crime Writers Association for the Debut Dagger shortlist which gave me the confidence to continue with it in the first place. Thanks also to Laura and all at Bedford Square/No Exit Press for picking the book up, and to Hannah, Polly, and the rest of the team for their subsequent hard work in getting it into shape and ready for publication.

Heartfelt thanks to my family, Laura, Will and Eleanor, for all their support and encouragement, with a special mention to my parents; the dysfunctional relationships in this book are most certainly not taken from personal experience. A big thanks to Tory for being there to vent to whenever needed, and always being a voice of reason. I'd also like to thank my NHS colleagues over the years, too many to name. The NHS remains an incredible institution, staffed by people who do a tough job for often very little reward, and in writing about dubious medical ethics for the purposes of fiction, it is not my intention to ever bring this dedication and hard work into question.

About the Author

C.J. Griffiths has spent most of his working life in the NHS, as a paramedic, anaesthetic practitioner and as part of a hospital resuscitation team. During his career he became fascinated with the unique level of trust involved in healthcare and was drawn to explore the darker side of medical ethics in his writing. He is the recipient of the Writers and Artists' Working-Class Writers Prize and was shortlisted for the CWA Debut Dagger Award. He lives in Buckinghamshire with his wife and children, and when not writing spends his time immersed in books, films and music.